NEUROLOGY - LABORATORY AND CLINICAL RESEARCH DEVELOPMENTS

PROGRESSIVE MULTIFOCAL LEUKOENCEPHALOPATHY

RISK FACTORS, MANAGEMENT STRATEGIES AND PROGNOSIS

Neurology - Laboratory and Clinical Research Developments

Additional books in this series can be found on Nova's website under the Series tab.

Additional e-books in this series can be found on Nova's website under the e-book tab.

NEUROLOGY - LABORATORY AND CLINICAL RESEARCH DEVELOPMENTS

PROGRESSIVE MULTIFOCAL LEUKOENCEPHALOPATHY

RISK FACTORS, MANAGEMENT STRATEGIES AND PROGNOSIS

DENISE S. COLEMAN
EDITOR

New York

Additional color graphics may be available in the e-book version of this book.

Library of Congress Cataloging-in-Publication Data

ISBN: 978-1-63482-889-5
Library of Congress Control Number: 2015939743

Published by Nova Science Publishers, Inc. † New York

CONTENTS

PREFACE

Progressive multifocal leukoencephalopathy (PML) is a rare, disabling and potentially fatal brain infection of the central nervous system (CNS) caused by reactivation of the John Cunningham virus (JCV). The most important risk factor for PML is immunosuppression associated with HIV/AIDS or therapy. Approximately 60 to 80% of the adult population has JC antibodies, but PML is rarely diagnosed. The chapters in this book include research on the pathologic features of PML, the diagnosis, risk factors, pathogenesis, and management strategies.

Chapter 1 - The John Cunningham virus (JCV) is a ubiquitous human polyomavirus affecting children or adolescents, remaining latent in the kidneys, bone marrow and lymphoid tissues. Due to genetic alterations in the virus, it is converted into a neurotropic prototype, which causes progressive demyelination in the CNS.

The most important risk factor for PML is immunosuppression associated with HIV/AIDS or therapy. In Multiple Sclerosis (MS), PML has been mostly associated with natalizumab, which not only prevents effective CNS immunosurveillance by JCV-specific T cells, but has also been associated with increasing peripheral expression of JCV. Biogen-sponsored data support a model of PML risk, which includes duration of treatment, JCV serology and history of prior immunosuppressive therapy.

The most common features in PML are neurobehavioural, motor, language, and visual perturbations. MRI lesions suggestive of PML should prompt a lumbar puncture (LP) and CSF JCV PCR using an ultrasensitive assay and, if workup including a negative second LP is unrevealing, a brain biopsy should be considered.

In MS patients, standard treatment for PML treatment is elimination of the drug from the bloodstream by plasma exchange or immune-adsorption techniques. In HIV-positive patients optimization of antiretroviral treatment is necessary. Other treatments such as antiviral agents, immunomodulatory and 5HT2A receptor antagonists have been tried without significant results.

After re-establishment of immunocompetence, almost all patients will develop immune reconstitution inflammatory syndrome (PML-IRIS), which is potentially disabling and fatal. The diagnosis of PML-IRIS is supported by MRI scans, and treatment consists of corticosteroids. In a few recent clinical reports, a T cell modulator maraviroc seemed to reduce PML-IRIS risk.

The mortality due to PML associated with natalizumab treatment has decreased over the years, with a survival rate greater than 70%, probably due to earlier detection and better understanding of the disease.

The most appropriate approach for PML is to avoid using natalizumab in MS patients with a high risk of developing PML, but if this risk is accepted in a very active disease, regular MRI and clinical vigilance is mandatory. In HIV-positive patients recovery of CD4 + T cell counts can offer a survival benefit.

Chapter 2 - Progressive multifocal leukoencephalopathy (PML) is a rare demyelinating disease of the central nervous system caused by infection of oligodendrocytes by a papovavirus, most commonly JC virus. It typically occurs in immunocompromised individuals. This chapter focuses on the pathologic features of PML, characterized by a histologic triad of demyelination, intranuclear inclusions within oligodendrocytes, and enlarged reactive astrocytes with irregular, hyperchromatic nuclei. The demyelination most commonly occurs in subcortical regions of the brain and typically spares the spinal cord. The pathologic diagnosis can be confirmed by immunohistochemistry, in-situ hybridization, polymerase chain reaction or electron microscopy. The authors also discuss the differential diagnosis of the histologic findings, including other demyelinating diseases such as multiple sclerosis, acute disseminated encephalomyelitis/postvaccineal encephalomyelitis and acute necrotizing hemorrhagic leukoencephalitis.

Chapter 3 - Progressive multifocal leukoencephalopathy (PML) is a neurological potencially fatal disease caused by JC polyomavirus, most often seen among patients with severe defects in the cellular immune system. Despite an 80% estimated seroprevalence of anti-JC virus antibodies in healthy people, development of symptoms in non-immunocompromised individuals is extremely rare.

Historically, this disease have gone through three big periods: in the early 1980s, PML was initially described in patients with lymphoproliferative diseases; with the acquired immune deficiency syndrome (AIDS) pandemic, PML affected 4-5% of all human immunodeficiency virus (HIV)-infected patients. Nowadays, after the development of antiretroviral therapy, and with the use of several monoclonal antibodies for cancer and autoimmune diseases, specially natalizumab-related multiple sclerosis, psoriasis treatment with efalizumab, and the widely use of rituximab, several cases have started to be more frequently described in these patients treated with these immunosupressants.

Typically, this infection will affect olygodendrocytes and their myelin processes, and symptoms will vary depending on the areas of demyelination. Its diagnosis will be confirmed after detection of viral DNA or proteins by in situ hybridation or by immunohistochemistry on a brain biopsy or after JC virus detection by a positive polymerase chain reaction (PCR) in the cerebrospinal fluid (CSF).

No treatment provided demonstrable therapeutic efficacy. Several clinical cases and small trials have been reported with different drugs including antineoplastic, immunomodulants, antiviral and antimalarial agents or serotoninergic antagonists; with many of the affected individuals dying from this disease. Because of all these failed efforts, immune reconstitution syndrome remains to be the most important and effective approach to treatment, with antiretrovirals as the standard therapy for HIV-patients and with worse outcome for non-HIV patients, since it is not always possible to withdraw their immunosupresive medication because of the risk.

Because PML still has today a high mortality rate, a development of treatments are urgently needed to impact in the survival of these individuals.

Chapter 4 - Progressive multifocal leukoencephalopathy (PML) is a debilitating and frequently fatal central nervous system demyelinating disease caused by JC virus (JCV), for which there is currently no effective treatment. Lytic infection of oligodendrocytes in the brain leads to their eventual destruction and progressive demyelination, resulting in multiple foci of lesions in the white matter of the brain. The recent advent of humanized monoclonal antibody therapy for the treatment of autoimmune inflammatory diseases such as multiple sclerosis and Crohn's disease has also led to an increased risk of PML as a side effect of immunotherapy. The authors would like to highlight the importance of a correct diagnostic assessment of the viral strain involved in the pathogenesis of PML, and the urgent need to identify possible risk factors and sensitive biomarkers detectable in the early phase of the disease. The study of JCV and the elucidation of the underlying causes of PML are important and active areas of research that may lead to new insights into immune function and host antiviral defense, as well as to potential new therapies. A combined approach with multiple compounds both interfering with different phases of the viral cycle and boosting specific components of the immune system involved in the response to JCV infection should be used.

Chapter 5 - The term "Immune reconstitution inflammatory syndrome" (IRIS) was originally introduced to describe the phenomenon of paradoxical clinical deterioration in HIV-infected patients despite the successful virological and immunological recovery after treatment with antiretroviral therapy.

This condition has actually been described even in the central nervous system (CNS) when immunosuppressed patients experience an opportunistic infection, as a result of an aberrant response of the immune function. Since new immunosuppressant therapies for autoimmune diseases or graft rejection in transplanted patients have been established, IRIS has become much more frequent, as a consequence of sudden immunosuppressive drug removal.

In Natalizumab treated multiple sclerosis (MS) patients, there is a well known risk of developing progressive multifocal encephalopathy (PML), a rare demyelinating disease of the subcortical white matter, requiring the reactivation of latent JCV reservoirs and the subsequent invasion of the CNS. PML typically presents with subacute neurological symptoms that mainly affect cognitive functions, with a progressive course sometimes leading to severe neurological deficits. When PML takes place the standard treatment is plasma exchange (PLEX) or immunoabsorption (IA). The drug removal from bloodstream restores lymphocyte trafficking into the CNS, leading to a massive infiltration into PML lesions.

Evidence from literature describes in nearly all cases of Natalizumab-associated PML the occurrence of IRIS, presenting as a subacute progression and exacerbation of earlier symptoms of PML within days to a few weeks after PLEX. PML-IRIS is the consequence of an enhanced immune response to disease-specific antigens, likely leading to an overproduction of inflammatory mediators.

This condition is differentiated in early or late PML-IRIS by the time course relative to PLEX/IA and contrast enhancement at the brain MRI. There is a variety of patterns of clinical presentation and evolution, ranging from asymptomatic to catastrophic.

The two major factors which contribute to the severity of IRIS are the degree of immune suppression and the rapidity of immune recovery. It has become routine so far to observe that a strong reactivation of the disease, in terms of inflammatory response, is a risk after the suspension of Natalizumab therapy in MS patients. The scientific community is now trying to differentiate the classical IRIS, typically occurring in the setting of PML, from the typical MS rebounds following Natalizumab suspension. Reports of outcomes after discontinuation of therapy suggested an eventual return of disease activity to pretreatment levels in terms of the degree of inflammatory response, which eventually increases with duration of therapy interruption.

In this chapter, the authors will focus on epidemiology, pathogenesis and treatment of IRIS with particular attention to cases following Natalizumab-associated PML.

In: Progressive Multifocal Leukoencephalopathy ISBN: 978-1-63482-889-5
Editor: Denise S. Coleman

Chapter 1

Progressive Multifocal Leukoencephalopathy: Current Concepts of a Renewed Disease

Inês Correia and Lívia Sousa
Neurology Department,
Centro Hospitalar e Universitário de Coimbra,
Portugal

Abstract

Progressive Multifocal Leukoencephalopathy (PML) is a rare, disabling and potentially fatal brain infection of the central nervous system (CNS) caused by reactivation of the John Cunningham virus (JCV). JCV is a ubiquitous human polyomavirus affecting children or adolescents, remaining latent in the kidneys, bone marrow and lymphoid tissues. Due to genetic alterations in the virus, it is converted into a neurotropic prototype, which causes progressive demyelination in the CNS.

The most important risk factor for PML is immunosuppression associated with HIV/AIDS or therapy. In Multiple Sclerosis (MS), PML has been mostly associated with natalizumab, which not only prevents effective CNS immunosurveillance by JCV-specific T cells, but has also been associated with increasing peripheral expression of JCV. Biogen-sponsored data support a model of PML risk, which includes duration of treatment, JCV serology and history of prior immunosuppressive therapy.

The most common features in PML are neurobehavioural, motor, language, and visual perturbations. MRI lesions suggestive of PML should prompt a lumbar puncture (LP) and CSF JCV PCR using an ultrasensitive assay and, if workup including a negative second LP is unrevealing, a brain biopsy should be considered.

In MS patients, standard treatment for PML treatment is elimination of the drug from the bloodstream by plasma exchange or immune-adsorption techniques. In HIV-positive patients optimization of antiretroviral treatment is necessary. Other treatments such as antiviral agents, immunomodulatory and 5HT2A receptor antagonists have been tried without significant results.

After re-establishment of immunocompetence, almost all patients will develop immune reconstitution inflammatory syndrome (PML-IRIS), which is potentially disabling and fatal. The diagnosis of PML-IRIS is supported by MRI scans, and treatment consists of corticosteroids. In a few recent clinical reports, a T cell modulator maraviroc seemed to reduce PML-IRIS risk.

The mortality due to PML associated with natalizumab treatment has decreased over the years, with a survival rate greater than 70%, probably due to earlier detection and better understanding of the disease.

The most appropriate approach for PML is to avoid using natalizumab in MS patients with a high risk of developing PML, but if this risk is accepted in a very active disease, regular MRI and clinical vigilance is mandatory. In HIV-positive patients recovery of CD4 + T cell counts can offer a survival benefit.

INTRODUCTION

Progressive Multifocal Leukoencephalopathy (PML) is a rare, disabling and potentially fatal brain infection of the central nervous system (CNS), caused by reactivation of the John Cunningham virus (JCV).

The most important risk factor for PML is the setting of immunosuppression associated with HIV/AIDS (HIV-PML), myeloproliferative diseases, or immunosuppressive therapy used in the treatment of multiple sclerosis (MS) and other autoimmune diseases.

In MS, PML has been mostly associated with natalizumab (natalizumab-PML), other treatments apparently not carrying the same risk of PML. Understanding how to manage PML risk in MS patients is one of the current goals in MS research. Since the underlying cause of PML is immunosuppression and there is no established antiviral treatment, PML-related care is based on immunocompetence re-institution.

In light of the current state of knowledge, the designation Progressive Multifocal Leukoencephalopathy is becoming obsolete, as PML is not a progressive disease in all cases, it can be just unifocal and grey matter may be involved making it more than a leukoencephalopathy.

This chapter will present a brief review of PML history, pathogenesis, pathology, risk factors, diagnosis and management, with a special focus on MS patients.

HISTORICAL REVIEW

The term PML was first introduced by Richardson, Astrom and Mancall in 1958. They described a rapidly progressive and fatal disease in two patients with chronic lymphocytic leukaemia, and in another with Hodgkin's disease. In the pathological studies, multifocal demyelination, nuclear enlargement, inclusions in oligodendrocytes and bizarre alterations of individual astrocytes were present. Considering these characteristics, these authors named the disease Progressive Multifocal Leukoencephalopathy.[1].

In 1961, Richardson recognized the association between PML and other immunosuppressed states, after studying cases associated with malignant lymphoma or leukaemia, carcinomatosis, miliar tuberculosis, sarcoidosis and advanced age [2]. The identification of inclusion bodies in the nuclei of damaged oligodendrocytes suggested that the disease might be related to a viral infection [2, 3]. This theory was confirmed in 1965 after the identification of large numbers of small virus-like particles resembling papova virions in PML glial nuclei [4, 5].

In 1971 the virus was isolated from the brain of a PML patient and received the patient's name – John Cunningham virus (JCV) [6].

PML remained a rare condition until the onset of the acquired immunodeficiency syndrome (AIDS) epidemic. Miller described the first case of HIV-PML in 1982, one year after the initial description of AIDS [7]. PML converted to a prominent opportunistic central nervous system infection and the incidence and reported deaths due to PML significantly increased from 0.15 cases per million people in 1974 to 0.61 cases per million in 1987 [8, 9]. Since highly active antiretroviral therapy – combined anti-retroviral treatment (cART) – became available, the incidence of PML has decreased significantly, the overall incidence of PML decreased from 14.8/1,000 patients per year in 1996 to 2.6 in 2005 and 0.8 in 2011 [10]. PML is currently considered one of the AIDS-defining illnesses in HIV-infected patients, with a prevalence of around 4-5% [11, 12, 13].

A study based on the Nationwide Inpatient Sample database from US reported a total of 9,675 cases of PML between 1998 and 2005, including 82% in AIDS, 8.4% in hematologic cancers, 2.8% in solid organ cancers and 0.4% with rheumatologic diseases [14].

PML has also been described in patients treated with several classes of medications which suppress the host's cellular immune response, such as in organ transplant recipients [14, 15].

Recently, a new category of PML patients has emerged among patients treated with monoclonal antibodies for autoimmune diseases [16].

PATHOGENESIS

JCV is a ubiquitous species-specific polyomavirus only found in humans and therefore, research on JC virus pathogenesis has been hampered by the lack of an animal model [17]. It is a small DNA polyomavirus with a 5.13 Kb enclosed circular double-stranded DNA (Figure 1). The enclosed circular genome is comprised of early and late coding (90% of the genome), which are encoded counterclockwise and clockwise, respectively, both controlled by a noncoding control region (NCCR) (10% of the genome). The early region is responsible for the expression of a series of proteins, named small and large T antigens, which possess regulatory functions in the viral replication cycle. The late region encodes three classes of structural proteins VP1, VP2, and VP3, which form the capsid of the virus, and agnoprotein (a protein necessary for DNA repair and cell cycle progression).

The JCV coding region for regulatory and structural proteins is largely conserved; it confers the genotype associated with the geographic origin of the patient and has not been convincingly associated with disease pathogenesis. However, the NCCR sequence of JCV is hypervariable and contains determinants for neurotropism and neurovirulence [17, 18].

To infect cells (Figure 2), JCV binds to the N-linked glycoprotein with an alpha (2,6)-linked sialic acid[19], which is present on many human cells, and to the serotoninergic 5HT2a receptor [17]. This receptor is present in several organs, such as the kidney, and in epithelial cells, B lymphocytes, platelets, glial cells and neurons [20, 21, 22].

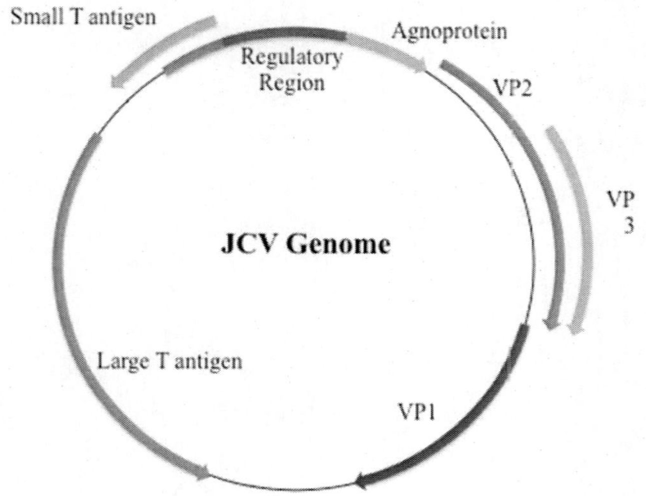

Figure 1. JCV Genome. Adapted from Tan et al. (2010) [17].

Pharmacological agents targeting the 5HT2a receptor have been shown to prevent infection of these cells in vitro [23]. JCV DNA has been detected in oligodendrocytes, astrocytes, lymphocytes [24], kidney epithelium cells, tonsil stromal cells [25] and plasma cells [26].

The primary infection generally occurs in childhood but serological studies indicate that it may also occur in adulthood [28, 29]. Following gastrointestinal or respiratory transmission [30, 31, 32], there is an invasion of the local lymphoid tissue and lymphocytes through which other parts of the body, such as bone marrow and the kidneys, become infected. After asymptomatic primary infection, the virus remains quiescent in the kidneys, bone marrow, and lymphoid tissue [25, 26, 33-35]. Occasionally, JC viremia may occur [36] and the virus can be intermittently excreted in the urine in 10–40% of adults [37-41].

The JCV NCCR most often detected in the urine has a stable sequence and is called the “archetype”, since it is considered to be the “wild-type” that is transmitted between individuals, from which all other forms have evolved (the archetype hypothesis) [42]. In opposition, the JCV NCCR most often isolated from the cerebrospinal fluid (CSF) and brain tissues of PML patients has rearrangements, including duplications, insertions, deletions and tandem repeats [18].

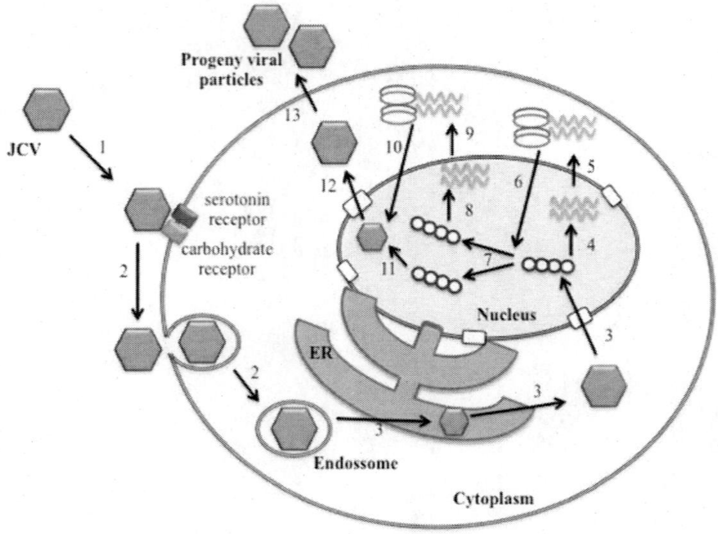

Figure 2. Life cycle and cellular events in JCV infection. 1: JCV binding to cellular surface sialic acid-linked carbohydrate receptor coupled to serotonin receptor. 2: Endocytosis of viral particle. 3: Onward translocation into the nucleus via the endoplasmic reticulum. In the nucleus the viral particle undergoes DNA replication, transcription and encapsulation. 4: Transcription of early viral coding region. 5: Translation of early mRNAs. 6: Nuclear relocalization. 7: Replication of viral particle. 8: Transcription of late viral coding region. 9: Translation of late viral transcript. 10: Nuclear localization of capsids. 11: Final nuclear packaging. 12: Intracellular release of viral particles. 13: Extracellular release of JCV progeny. Adapted from Adiele et al. 2014 [27].

Sequence rearrangement from the "archetype" to the "neurotropic" type may increase restricted tissue tropism or virulence, therefore affecting the overall pathogenic potential of the virus [43].

Recently, a study using deep sequencing to perform a JC virus quasispecies analysis of NCCR DNA, amplified from body fluid samples from PML patients, revealed a complex mixture composed of multiple viral variants suggestive of a highly dynamic process of JCV NCCR reorganization in vivo. It also suggested viral dissemination towards the brain via the haematogenous route [44]. PML occurs when JCV is unchecked by cellular immunity, is reactivated, and migrates to the CNS where it infects glial cells [17]. The rarity of PML despite the widespread prevalence of JCV infection in the world's population implies that there are multiple barriers to the development of the disease. A significant predisposing factor for the development of PML is cell-mediated immune dysfunction, since a rearranged NCCR necessary for reactivation of JC virus resulting in PML arises in the context of immunosuppression [17]. In this setting, not only will increased viral multiplication contribute to dissemination of the viral particle and formation of lesions associated with PML, but also the depressed immune system will be unable to react against the infection and promote clearance of the viral particles [45]. Moreover, monoclonal antibody therapeutic agents prevent translocation of T lymphocytes through the blood-brain barrier, resulting in reduction of T cell-linked immunosurveillance [46].

Studies involving HIV-PML [47] and natalizumab-PML [48] have largely contributed to shedding light on the immune mechanism against JCV; it has been described as an extremely inflammatory cellular infiltrate with a majority of CD8+ T cells aggregating around infected oligodendrocytes, accompanied by CD20+ B cells and CD138+ plasma cells.

Early after disease onset, JCV-specific CD8+ T-cell responses were significantly higher in PML survivors than non-surviving PML patients and this apparently constitutes a valuable prognostic marker of disease evolution [49, 50]. Conversely, almost half of non-surviving PML patients had detectable JCV-specific CD4+ T cells, which did not prevent a fatal outcome [50]. Antibody-mediated immunity does not protect against PML as patients with a high JCV index are not only unprotected from PML but are also apparently at higher risk of developing this disease [51].

PATHOLOGY

JCV promotes a lytic infection of oligodendrocytes, leading to massive destruction of myelin sheaths (Figure 3). The typical findings in PML lesions are oligodendrocytes with enlarged nuclei containing JCV inclusions, occasionally accompanied by distorted astrocytes. With hematoxylin–eosin (HE) staining, the viral inclusions appear as amphophilic material dispersed throughout the nucleoplasm (full inclusions) (Figure 4). Nevertheless, numerous cells with a clearer nucleoplasm and marginated chromatin are also seen, but lacking amphophilic material despite nuclear enlargement [52].

The presence of JCV is confirmed by immunohistochemistry, in situ nucleic acid hybridization, or electron microscopy [53]. Some studies have shown that JCV also infects neurons in cerebellar granule layers and pyramidal neurons in the cerebral cortex[54-56], which explains the frequent severe disability after PML.

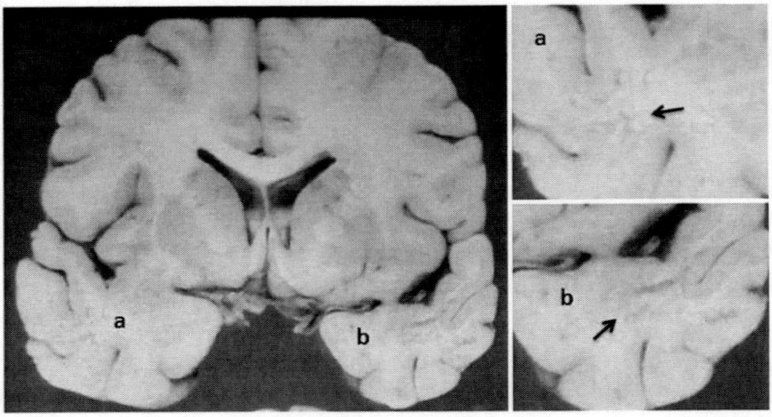

Figure 3. PML patient brain autopsy. Macroscopy revealed characteristic gross appearance of PML with multiple irregularly demarcated subcortical demyelination foci (arrows, magnification in a and b).

The degree of demyelination and inflammation is variable in localization and evolution over time. In some samples there is only myelin pallor whereas others show marked degeneration associated with axonal damage and numerous foamy macrophages harboring phagocytolytic lipids or myelin debris. The latter lesions, often observed in cases associated with AIDS, are regarded as "burnt out" lesions [57, 58].

In PML the inflammatory response is usually poor, contrasting with IRIS, where severe inflammatory and demyelinating lesions with marked infiltration by macrophages and CD8 T lymphocytes are usually present [59-64].

Risk Factors

The most important risk factor for PML is the setting of immunosuppression inherent to AIDS, but also related to treatment of inflammatory diseases including MS, Rheumatoid Arthritis, Systemic Lupus Erythematosus and Sarcoidosis [27].

AIDS

In HIV patients, CD4+ and CD8+ T lymphopenia is the primary PML risk factor.

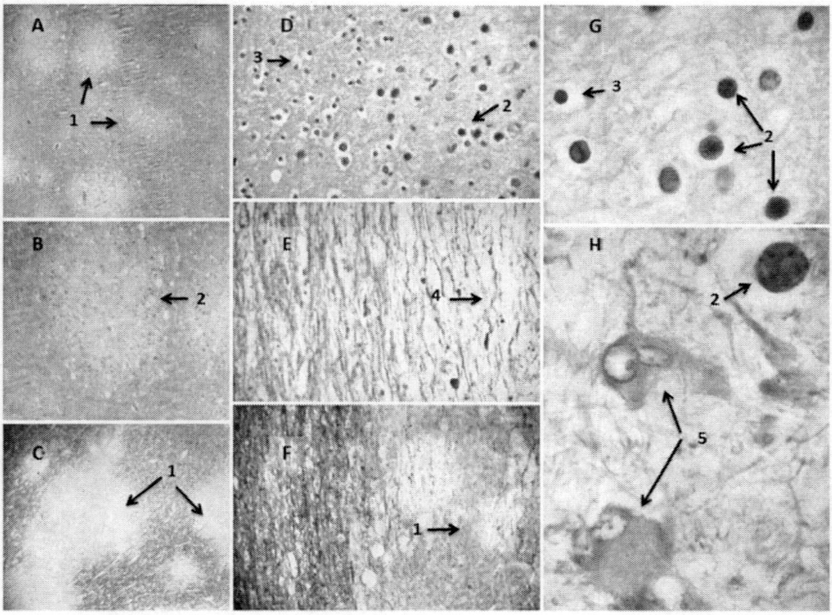

Figure 4. Neuropathology of progressive multifocal Leukoencephalopathy. A - Broad myelin pallor in the white matter (arrow 1) (hematoxylin–eosin (HE) staining). B – Magnification of the previous image, with enlarged oligodendrocytes visible in the periphery of the lesion (arrow 2) (HE staining). C – Small well-demarcated lesions fuse to form larger lesions (arrow 1, Kluver-Barrera (KB) staining). D and G – oligodendrocytes with enlarged nuclei containing amphophilic inclusions dispersed throughout the nucleoplasm (arrow 2) on the side of the lesion; normal oligodendrocytes (arrow 3) (HE staining). E – rarefaction of axons in the lesion (arrow 4, Glisen staining). F – myelin pallor in the lesion (arrow 1, KB staining). H – oligodendrocytes harboring amphophilic inclusions in the enlarged nuclei (arrow 2); distorted astrocytes (arrow 5) (GFAP staining).

In a recent study published in 2014 the median CD4+ cell count at diagnosis was 82 cells/mm3; 39% had a CD4+ count above 100 cells/mm3 and 13% above 200 cells/mm3 [10].

Although the use of c-ART markedly improves immune function and prognosis in HIV-infected patients [65], PML may develop or worsen with antiretroviral therapy despite a recovery of the immune system – this is called Immune Reconstitution Inflammatory Syndrome (PML-IRIS). When it presents after the initiation of cART as an exacerbation of already established PML it is defined as “paradoxical worsening” PML-IRIS, otherwise as “unmasking” PML-IRIS [59-64, 66-82]. In a case report series, 18% of patients with PML experienced an exacerbation – PML-IRIS – within the first nine weeks of cART, associated with a reduction in the plasma HIV RNA level and an increased CD4 T-cell count [83].

Multiple Sclerosis

The first two natalizumab-PML cases were described in 2005 in the SENTINEL Trial, were natalizumab was an add-on to Interferon beta-1a [84, 85]. A third PML case was also reported in a Crohn's disease patient treated with natalizumab, who hade been previously exposed to azathioprine. These reports were attributed to the association of natalizumab with other drugs and natalizumab sales in the US were suspended for investigation [86]. After 16 months of market withdrawal, the drug was reintroduced as an approved MS treatment in monotherapy [87].

However, over 500 MS confirmed natalizumab-PML cases have been reported in approximately 132,600 patients exposed to natalizumab in the post-marketing setting worldwide [88].

Natalizumab is a humanized monoclonal antibody against alpha 4-integrin, designed to physically interfere with the binding of very late activating antigen 4 (VLA-4) on leukocytes to its natural fibronectin and vascular cell adhesion molecule-1 (VCAM-1) on the luminal surface of blood vessels.

Consequently, leukocytes are impaired in their ability to migrate from peripheral blood into other tissues and are destined to spend most of their life cycle within the circulation [89]. Several reasons have been put forward to explain the increased risk of PML associated with natalizumab.

Natalizumab prevents effective CNS immunosurveillance by JCV-specific T cells by blocking alpha-4 beta-1 integrin and leads to changes in CSF CD4/CD8 ratios, similar to those seen in HIV infection, for up to 6 months. Although CD4/CD8 ratios in peripheral blood in patients with MS progressively decreased with the number of natalizumab doses, they remained within normal limits [90, 91]. These findings seem to be related to the lower expression of unbound α4-integrin, pre and post-natalizumab therapy, of CD4+ T compared to CD8+ T cells, since the unbound fraction of VLA-4 on the cell surface remains available for the cell to adhere to biological membranes and to migrate into peripheral tissues [90].

In addition, treatment with natalizumab seems to prompt profound T-cell receptor repertoire restrictions in the CSF, which reflects an altered immune surveillance of the CNS, and is associated with impaired or delayed peripheral expansion of antigen-specific T cells [92].

Besides an altered immune surveillance of the CNS, natalizumab has been implicated in changes of JCV replication. An increase in ongoing JCV replication was suspected in a study where a time-related increase in JC virus-specific effector memory T cells was demonstrated in natalizumab patients [93]. In addition, in 19 MS patients, JC viruria was detected in baseline samples in 19% of the cases, but 12 months after natalizumab treatment this number increased to 63%. It was also found that after natalizumab treatment, blood samples and most of the urine samples had NCCRs similar to those usually found in PML, the neurotropic prototype virus. Furthermore, a drop in immunity against JCV was shown, starting after 6 months of natalizumab treatment[94], which may contribute to an impaired response to the virus.

Concerns regarding JCV dissemination have also been raised with natalizumab treatment. Natalizumab has been associated with an increased release of CD34+ hematopoietic precursors from bone marrow [91, 95-97]. These precursors have been implicated in the dissemination of JCV because JCV DNA has been detected in them [98, 99], although this was not observed in other studies [100, 101]. Natalizumab has also been shown to reduce the retention of T, NK and B cells in secondary lymphoid organs, inducing a chronic and maintained increase in peripheral blood, and memory B cells may act as carriers of neurotropic JCV variants to the brain [91].

Industry-sponsored data support a model of PML risk, which includes JCV serology, treatment for longer than 2 years and a history of prior immunosuppressive therapy (Table 1) [102]. When all of these factors are present, the risk of developing PML is estimated to be about 1% [103-105].

In a large multinational MS cohort including 10,280 patients, the overall anti-JCV antibody prevalence was 57.6%, ranging from 47.4% in Norway to 67.7% in Turkey [29].

Seronegative patients are at low risk of PML, but repeated measurements of the anti-JCV antibody titer are necessary to exclude the possibility of seroconversion during treatment [105]. Apparently, there is a continuum of PML risk in patients with no prior immunosuppressant treatment, which is predicted by the anti-JCV antibody index, as reported in a study from Plavina et al. (2014), including 71 natalizumab-treated PML patients and 2522 non-PML JCV seropositive (JCV+) patients. Patients with an index below 1.5 during the first 24 months had a PML risk similar to that for anti-JCV antibody–negative patients (0.1/1,000).

Table 1. PML Risk Estimates per 1,000 Patients by Anti-JCV Antibody Status

Negative	Positive					
	Natalizumab Exposure (months)	Prior IS Use	No Prior IS Use (According to JCV-ab index)			
			≤0.9	≤1.1	≤1.5	>1.5
<0.1	1–24	1.8	0.1	0.1	0.1	1.0
	25–48	11.2	0.3	0.7	1.2	8.1
	49–72	Insufficient data	0.4	0.7	1.3	8.5

PML = Progressive Multifocal Leukoencephalopathy; IS = Immunosuppressive treatment; JCV-ab = JCV antibody. Adapted from Plavina et al. 2013 [51] and Biogen Idec data available online.

Between month 25 and 72 the risk ranged from 0.3 to 1.3/1,000. Patients with an index above 1.5 had a PML risk of 1/1,000 during the first 24 months, and eight times greater between months 25 to 72. Otherwise, 96% of the patients who developed PML persistently had an index above 0.9 several months before PML [51].

The other factor associated with increased PML risk in natalizumab patients is prior immunosuppression [102], since 38% of the natalizumab-PML patients had been previously treated with immunosuppressive agents, including mitoxantrone, azathioprine, methotrexate, cyclophosphamide, or mycophenolate. Based on these observations, the estimated risk of PML in this group of patients was three to fourfold greater than that in patients who did not use immunosuppressant therapy before natalizumab therapy. The authors proposed that immunosuppressive drugs could contribute to long-term changes in the immune system and be involved in JCV mutation, which would explain the increased risk of PML even after a long interval between the exposure to the immunosuppressive drugs and natalizumab therapy [106]. In patients with previous immunosuppressive treatment the index is not a valid tool since there were no differences between patients who did or did not develop PML, although all PML patients were JCV+ [51].

Several studies have focused on finding other factors that can contribute to PML risk stratification. A low percentage expression of L-selectin on CD4+ T cells has been associated with an increased PML risk in both AIDS [107] and MS patients treated with natalizumab [108]. In a study published in 2015, JCV+ patients with lipid-specific immunoglobulin M oligoclonal (IgM) bands in the cerebrospinal fluid had reduced levels of PML risk similar to patients who were anti-JC negative, and a higher risk was observed in JCV+ patients negative for IgM bands [109].

In MS patients, PML has been mostly associated with natalizumab, and the other treatments such as fingolimod, dimethyl fumarate or alemtuzumab do not carry the same risk of PML [102], although some cases have been reported.

Fingolimod is a sphingosine 1-phosphate receptor modulator that reversibly redistributes lymphocytes into lymphoid tissue, whilst preserving lymphocyte function [110]. A few cases of PML have been reported in MS patients treated with fingolimod after natalizumab [111-113], and recently a case without previous immunosuppression or natalizumab treatment has been reported [114].

Others Immunosuppressive Treatments

A study conducted by Schmedt in 2012, which included 635 PML cases in approximately 2 million patients treated with immunosuppressive drugs, confirmed a higher risk of PML development not only with the monoclonal antibodies natalizumab, rituximab and efalizumab, but also with mycophenolate mofetil, tacrolimus and possibly with azathioprine, cyclosporine and cyclophosphamide [87].

Rituximab is a chimeric IgG1 monoclonal antibody that targets CD20+ B lymphocytes for lysis and depletion from the peripheral circulation. It is approved for treatment in CD20+ non-Hodgkin lymphoma, and is also used in conjunction with methotrexate for the reduction of symptoms in patients with rheumatoid arthritis for whom treatment with tumor necrosis factor-alpha inhibitors has previously failed, and more recently in lupus, and off-label in demyelinating diseases such as Neuromyelitis Optica. 114 PML cases have been reported in association with rituximab, although none in patients with demyelinating diseases [115]. However, it is difficult to isolate its role in the development of PML because most of these patients had lymphoproliferative diseases and had previously received several other classes of immunosuppressive drugs [17].

CLINICAL MANIFESTATIONS

PML is usually a subacute process, progressing over days to weeks, with an insidious onset but with a fast disability accumulation [116]. The neurological impairment in PML is determined by the location, size and distribution of PML lesions in the brain.

The most frequently affected regions are the frontal, parietal and occipital lobes. The deep gray structures, cerebellum and brainstem may also be involved. The spine is rarely affected [76, 117-119].

The most frequently reported manifestations are neurobehavioural dysfunction and cognitive impairment (49%), motor deficits (hemiparesis or apraxia, 37%), speech impairment (dysarthria or aphasia, 31%), visual disturbances (hemianopsia, 26%), cerebellar dysfunction (ataxia, 17%), and sensory deficits (sensory loss or neglect, 3%) [105].

Seizures, both focal or generalized, may present in different phases of the disease evolution, from the first clinical manifestation of the disease, in PML-IRIS or as a disease sequel. In the first studies seizures were reported in 18% of the cases, but recent studies have shown seizures to be present in 36 to 53% of natalizumab-PML cases. This is an indication of gray matter involvement, which is associated with demyelinating lesions immediately adjacent to the cortex [120-125].

Headache and diplopia are less frequent [126, 127]. The disease is usually multi-symptomatic, but a single neurological abnormality at onset may be the only clinical and radiological manifestation [128].

When the immune system is restored and the subsequent response to antigens exacerbates the PML pathology, a paradoxical worsening of the disease, defined as PML-IRIS, may occur after some days to a few weeks. This entity is very relevant, since the exacerbation may be responsible for rostrocaudal deterioration of the patient with stupor and coma, occasionally complicated by respiratory arrest, warranting intensive care and invasive ventilator support [129, 130]. It is usually more aggressive in natalizumab-PML patients than those with HIV-PML because in the former case the immune system is generally intact after removal of the drug [123]. Although there are some reports of patients making a good recovery, most of those who survive may become very disabled with a high Expanded Disability Status

Scale (EDSS) score, and the recovery time may last several months. In a case series with 28 natalizumab-PML cases, 8 patients died, all of them in the PML-IRIS phase [123].

Other clinical entities have been associated with JCV infection. Involvement of granule cell neurons in the cerebellum leads to JCV Granule Cell Neuronopathy, which can occur in isolation or concomitantly with PML. Clinically, there is a subacute or chronic onset of cerebellar dysfunction, including ataxia and dysarthria [54, 131, 132].

The real incidence of JCV Granule Cell Neuronopathy is not known, but in a histological survey of brain samples from 43 patients known to have PML, up to 51% of them also had JCV-infected granule cell neurons [55]. Some reports of meningitis associated with JCV have been reported, even in immunocompetent patients [133-135].

INVESTIGATION

Any new neurological symptom or sign in patients at risk of developing PML should raise suspicions in order to avoid a delay in diagnosis [123].

The diagnosis of PML is achieved by combining the clinical presentation with diagnostic imaging techniques, laboratory tests and possibly a biopsy [17].

The algorithm for diagnosing PML is presented in Figure 5.

Imaging

Brain Magnetic Resonance Imaging (MRI) is the radiological modality of choice in diagnosing PML and screening patients at risk for PML, as it can detect early-stage lesions, even before they are clinically detectable [116].

On MRI (Table 2, Figure 4 and 5) the lesions are hyperintense on T2-weighted and fluid attenuated inversion recovery (FLAIR) images and hypointense on T1-weighted images[17], occasionally with microcystic changes. These lesions are sometimes more prominent on DWI imaging due to T2 "shine through" [102].

Multiple lesions may be present. They are confluent, usually greater than 3 cm, and mostly located in the the arcuate fibers (U fibers) between the cortex and white matter, with distinct borders next to gray matter and ill-defined borders next to white matter.

Lesions have also been described in the cerebellar peduncles and grey matter structures such as the basal ganglia or thalamus, where myelinated fibers reside [17, 116, 136]. Typical lesions do not respect any vascular territory and are usually devoid of oedema or mass effect on imaging [17, 136].

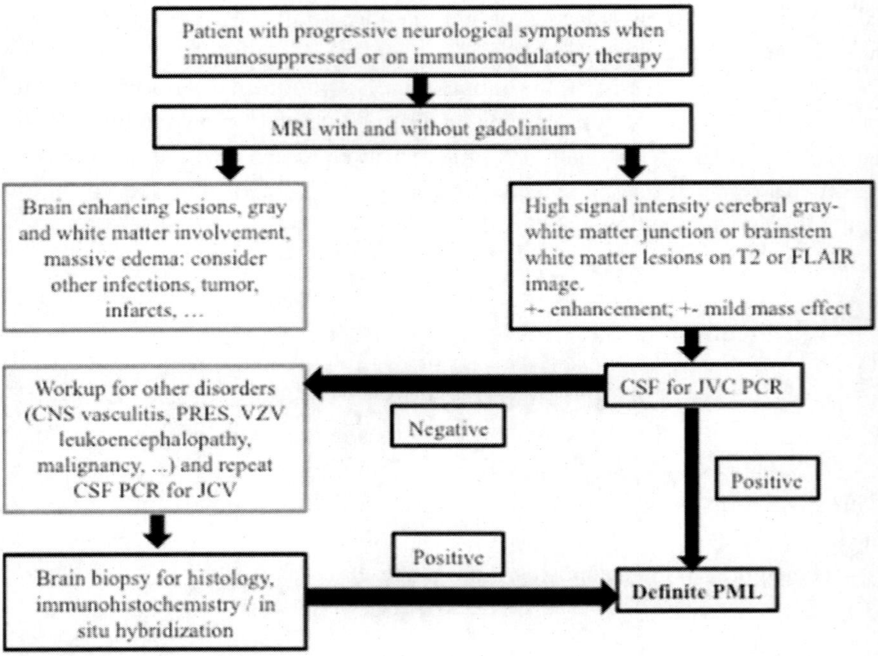

FLAIR = fluid-attenuated inversion recovery; JCV = JC virus; PML = progressive multifocal leukoencephalopathy; PRES = posterior reversible encephalopathy syndrome; VZV = varicella-zoster virus. Adapted from Berger et al., 2013 [128].

Figure 5. Algorithm for diagnosing progressive multifocal leukoencephalopathy.

In a revision of 40 PML patients associated with natalizumab, all lesions had a subcortical location, which was attributed to the presence of high blood flow, and there was cortical involvement in more than 50% of the cases [48, 136]. Approximately 40% of natalizumab-PML patients have lesions presenting Gadolinium enhancement [123] compared to only approximately 15% of HIV-PML patients [126]. Gadolinium enhancement is usually sparse, with a thin or reticulated appearance adjacent on to the edge of the lesions [102, 124]. Advanced PML is associated with an increased size and confluence of lesions, involvement of other areas, varying degrees of cortical atrophy and ventricular dilatation [116, 120]. MRI spectroscopy studies of PML lesions have reported decreased N-acetylaspartate, increased lactate and myoinositol, less frequently an increase in choline and occasionally an increase in lipids [137, 138].

The differential diagnosis of PML is extensive, particularly in HIV patients, and includes HIV encephalopathy, cytomegalovirus infection, varicella-zoster leukoencephalitis, MS-like illness, acute disseminated encephalomyelitis, CNS vasculitis, reversible leukoencephalopathy associated with nucleoside analogue antiretrovirals, white matter oedema associated with primary or metastatic brain tumours and CD8 encephalitis [128, 139].

In MS patients, it is extremely important and particularly difficult to differentiate PML lesions from new MS lesions. While the classic images of MS lesions are rounded well-circumscribed T2 lesions, occasionally associated with open-ring enhancement with minimal mass effect, PML lesions tend to be larger, confluent and subcortical, with an ill-defined border toward the white matter and sharp border towards the grey matter, and with punctate T2 hyperintensities in the area surrounding the PML lesions in approximately 70% of cases [102, 136, 139].

PML-IRIS should be suspected when mass effect and enhancement are more prominent, particularly if accompanied by a clinical deterioration. Due to the local inflammation and breakdown of the blood-brain barrier, oedema, swelling, mass effect, brain herniation and death may occur [59, 61, 63, 64, 66, 67, 69, 71, 75, 77, 102]. Brain Computed Tomography (CT) may be used but it is a less sensitive imaging method than MRI [17, 140]. On CT the lesions are hypodense or patchy.

Laboratory Tests

The increased risk of PML is associated with the presence of anti-JCV antibodies, currently detected and quantified by the second-generation STRATIFY JCV test [51]. In the right clinical context, an MRI suggestive of PML should prompt a lumbar puncture, since the diagnosis of PML is established by detection of JCV DNA in CSF by polymerase chain reaction (PCR) using an ultrasensitive assay [17], and it helps in excluding other diagnoses [128]. The ability to detect JCV is related to the sensitivity of the quantitative PCR techniques and on cART [124]. Previous to the cART era, the detection of JCV by PCR had a specificity and sensitivity above 90%, which dropped to 58% after the introduction of cART [124]. With the development of ultrasensitive PCR techniques, the sensitivity to detect JCV in CSF rose to above 95% [128], although a negative result does not entirely exclude PML, since in HIV patients under cART, MS patients and other autoimmune disease patients, the viral loads are often low and more likely to induce false negative results [128].

Table 2. Imaging features of Multiple Sclerosis, PML and PML-IRIS

	Multiple Sclerosis	PML	PML-IRIS
Size in T2 / FLAIR sequences	<3 cm	Usually >3 cm	Dependent on previous PML extension
Distribution	Periventricular, juxtacortical, infratentorial	Subcortical at gray-white junction, peripheral, infratentorial	
Shape	Rounded	Amorphous, following white matter tracts	
Borders	Well circumscribed	Distinct borders next to gray matter and ill-defined next to white matter	
Mass Effect	Mild	None	Significant
T1 Sequence	T1 hypointense (black holes)	Patchy T1 hypointensity	Occasionally rim of T1 hyperintensity
Gadolinium Enhancement	Well-defined borders, open ring enhancement	Variable, speckled or nodular patterns	More pronounced
Diffusion Sequences	Sometimes ADC hypointense with DWI hyperintensity	DWI bright due to T2 “shine through” – helps in differentiating PML lesions from chronic MS lesions	
Evolution	Variable	Rapid enlargement and extension along white matter tracts	Variable

Notes: PML = Progressive Multifocal Leukoencephalopathy; PML-IRIS: PML-Immune Reconstitution Inflammatory Syndrome. Adapted from Carruthers et al. 2013 [102].

The CSF PCR for JCV may be negative in PML-IRIS patients since the recovering immune system is able to partially contain viral replication to a level below the detection threshold of the PCR assay [17].

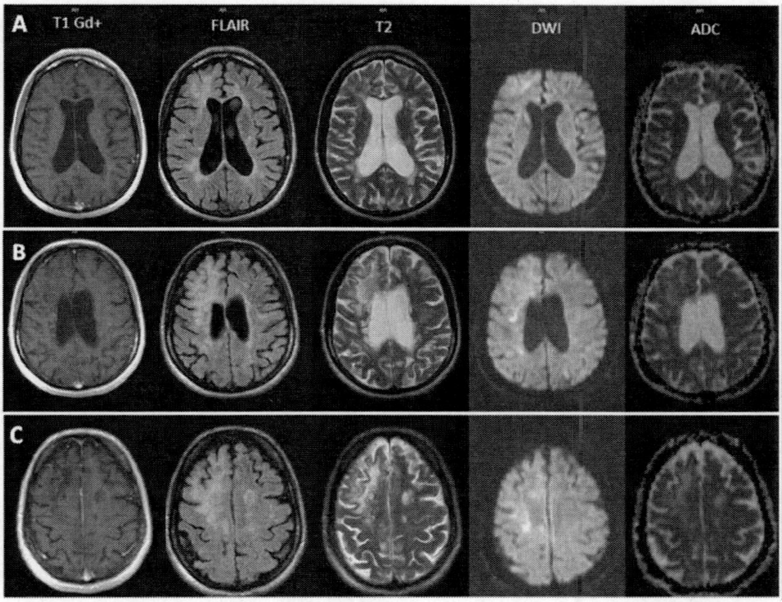

Figure 6. PML in a 35-year-old female patient treated with natalizumab for 66 months. Previous EDSS 6.5. A: PML (EDSS 7.5); B: PML-IRIS (EDSS 8.0); C: brain MRI 2 years after PML-IRIS (EDSS 8.0, hemiplegia, dysarthria and dementia).

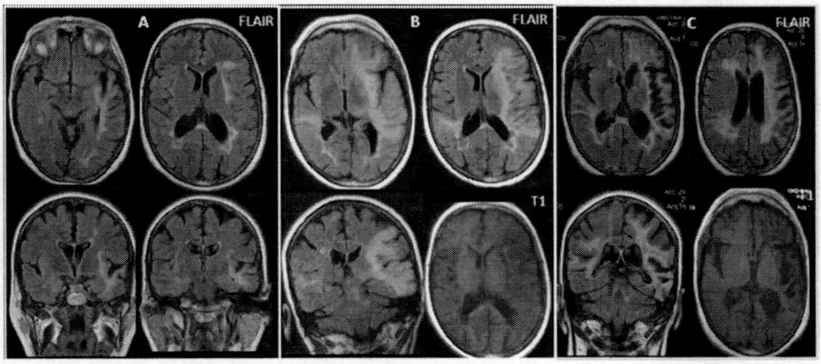

Figure 7. PML in a 50-year-old female patient treated with natalizumab for 28 months. A: PML (EDSS 4.0, previous EDSS 1.5); B: severe PML-IRIS after one month (EDSS 9.0); C: brain MRI six months after PML-IRIS (EDSS 7.0, hemiparesis, aphasia, moderate cognitive impairment).

CSF cell counts are usually less than 20 cells/mm3, and occasionally there is elevated CSF protein and rarely hypoglycorrhachia[126].

Pathology

A brain biopsy should be considered if the previous workup is unrevealing.

Diagnostic Criteria

According to the diagnostic criteria published by the American Academy of Neurology Neuroinfectious Disease Section for PML in 2013, PML can be definitive, probable, or possible, based on a combination of factors with or without pathological confirmation (Table 3) [128].

Management Strategies

Treatment for PML should begin immediately upon clinical suspicion, and should not be delayed for confirmatory laboratory testing or imaging.

Currently there are no specific anti-JCV infection treatments, and the best therapeutic option is to restore the immune system. Therefore, in patients with PML, the cause of underlying immunosuppression must be addressed and it is important to be aware of the possibility of PML-IRIS, since it can be destructive if unchecked [17, 102, 124].

HIV-PML

The prognosis of PML in HIV patients is improved by cART because it reduces the retroviral load in most body fluids and increases the number of CD4 T cells [53, 124].

The recommendations of the Center for Disease Control, National Institutes of Health and the HIV Medicine Association of the Infectious Diseases Society of America vary, depending on the patient's antiretroviral treatment status and its efficacy. cART should be started immediately in patients who have PML and who are not on therapy. If patients are already on therapy but remain HIV-viremic because of antiretroviral resistance, their cART regimen should be optimized. The approach in patients who develop PML despite successful virological suppression while taking cART is more complicated, and although an ART-intensification strategy with four classes of ART is a possibility, its effectiveness requires further studies [53, 124].

Natalizumab-PML

In HIV-negative patients the standard PML treatment is elimination of potential sources of immunosuppression from the bloodstream by plasma exchange (PLEX) or immune-adsorption techniques (IA) [17, 102, 124].

Table 3. PML Diagnostic Criteria

PML diagnosis without histopathology			
Certainty of PML diagnosis	Compatible clinical features	Compatible imaging findings	CSF PCR for JCV
Definite	+	+	+
Probable	+	-	+
	-	+	+
Possible	+	+	-/ND
	-	-	+
Certainty of PML diagnosis	Classic histopathologic triad	Immunohisto-chemistry or electron microscopy	Tissue PCR for JCV
Definite	+	+	+
	+	-/ND	+
	+	+	-/ND
Probable	+	-	-/ND
Possible	-	+	-/ND
Not PML	-	-	-/ND

Abbreviations: PML = Progressive Multifocal Leukoencephalopathy; ND = not done; PCR = polymerase chain reaction; + = positive; - = negative.

Classic histopathologic triad: demyelination, bizarre astrocytes, enlarged oligodendroglial nuclei.

Adapted from Berger et al. 2013[128].

In MS patients with natalizumab-PML, suspension of natalizumab and plasma removal of the drug as early as possible is the essential step in the treatment of PML. PLEX and IA accelerate clearance of natalizumab and desaturation of alpha4-integrin [17, 102, 124]. Restoration of leukocyte transmigratory capacity occurs when plasma concentration of natalizumab is less than 1 μg/ml, usually 15 days after three sessions of PLEX or at 82 days without PLEX [141, 142]. Although PLEX and/or IA is recommended, it is not mandatory and some authors suggest that it may be reasonable to hold plasma exchange in patients who develop PML after more than 55 days since the last natalizumab infusion (5 half-lives) [102].

Removal of the medication leads to effective immune reconstitution, but this rapid correction in immunosuppression can lead to immune reconstitution inflammatory syndrome, typically observed 2–6 weeks later [105].

In a study published in 2011 which included 42 cases of PML related to natalizumab treatment, most patients had 3–5 sessions of PLEX/IA, administered on alternate days with 1–1.5 times plasma volumes in each exchange. All patients initially improved or stabilized with the withdrawal of natalizumab and PLEX/IA, but paradoxically worsened subsequently, with the development of IRIS-PML; it seemed moreover that PLEX/IA had accelerated IRIS [143].

In a study published in 2013 with 15 cases of PML related to natalizumab, all patients received PLEX and/or IA to re-establish an immune response (5 only received PLEX, 1 only received immunoadsorption and 9 patients received both treatments), associated with supportive therapy with mefloquine and mirtazapine. All patients showed initial improvement or stabilisation in the weeks after PLEX and/or IA, but 14 of the 15 patients later developed IRIS, although there were no fatal cases recorded [144].

Some patients were treated with corticosteroids at the initial presentation of PML when their symptoms were mistaken for an MS relapse, but the early use of corticosteroids had no impact on the eventual outcome in this group [143].

Numerous treatments have been used taking into account the life cycle of JCV and the pathogenesis of PML, such as antiviral agents (cytarabine, cidofovir or topotecan), immunomodulatory therapies (interferon alfa, interferon beta, interleukin-2), hematopoietic growth factors (IL-7), 5HT2a receptor antagonists (risperidone, mirtazapine, chlorpromazine, mefloquine) and intravenous immunoglobulins, although there is no solid evidence of their usefulness in vivo [27, 145]. The first antiviral therapy tried in PML was cytarabine in 1974 [146], but it was later shown to be ineffective in an open-label randomized multicenter clinical trial for HIV-PML [147]. In 1998 cidofovir was tested in PML but a meta-analysis published in 2008 failed to identify a survival benefit in HIV-PML [148]. Topotecan was beneficial in 3 of 11 HIV-PML patients included in an uncontrolled and unblinded trial, but moderately severe or severe haematological changes were documented in more than 40% of the patients [149].

Interferon-alpha was beneficial in HIV-PML in one non-randomized and uncontrolled open-label observational study published in 1998 [150] but a later retrospective analysis failed to demonstrate any benefit beyond that conferred by cART alone in HIV-PML [151]. Treatment with beta-interferon, an inhibitor of viral replication, yielded variable results [152]. Interleukin-2 has been shown to lead to an increase in T-cell counts, thereby increasing the probability of immune control of JCV infection. Anecdotal reports of Interleukin-2 treatment in PML have been published [153-155], but no benefit was confirmed in two large trials (no benefit in survival or against opportunistic diseases in HIV patients) [156].

Interleukin-7 associated with JCV capsid protein VP1, and Toll-like receptor 7 agonist as adjuvant have been used in 2 PML cases not associated with HIV, with apparent benefit [157].

Since the 5-HT2A serotonin receptor has been found to act as a receptor for JCV in glial cells [23], several trials of drugs with a 5-HT2a receptor antagonist effect, such as risperidone [158] or mirtazapine [159], have been attempted. Mirtazapine has been used anecdotally at 15 mg/d to 30 mg/d as add-on to other agents, including cytosine arabinoside and cidofovir, and after alteration of their immunosuppressive regimen, in patients with non-HIV related PML, but no consistent results have been achieved so far [143, 160, 161]. It has been suggested that risperidone is potentially more powerful [162]. No controlled trials of 5-HT2a receptor antagonists in PML have been performed, although no significant effect on survival was noted with mirtazapine in one prospective study of the determinants of survival in PML [163]. Chlorpromazine [164] was also tried, due to its inhibition of clathrin-dependent endocytosis required for viral infection, but it had little or no benefit in a clinical trial in vivo [164].

In 2009 approximately two thousand already known drugs were screened and tested for activity against JCV in an in vitro JCV infection assay. 14 drug candidates with in vitro anti-JCV activity were identified and, of those, only mefloquine, an antimalarial agent, could inhibit the replication of JCV when applied in concentrations that had previously been documented to accumulate in the CNS of patients treated for malaria [165]. Apparently, it works by inhibiting JCV replication in cells after viral entry, even JCV strains typically causing PML [165], and several case reports have been published so far [129, 143, 166-168].

An open-label and randomized study with 37 PML patients evaluated the effect of mefloquine (250 mg/d for 3 days, then 250 mg weekly), but this study was terminated prematurely since preplanned interim data analyses suggested that there was no benefit on any outcome measure including CSF viral load, neuroimaging, clinical efficacy measure, survival duration and mortality [169].

In the absence of standard recommendations regarding specific anti-JCV infection treatments and the lack of plentiful high quality data, physicians may offer medicines such as mefloquine and mirtazapine on a case-by-case basis [102].

PML-IRIS

In patients with a reversible cause of immunosuppression, re-establishment of immunocompetence can be associated with PML-IRIS, which consists of an exuberant inflammatory response against JCV [66, 67, 102]. This immune reconstitution is secondary to an increase in T-lymphocyte counts, which usually follows the commencement of cART in HIV patients, or after cessation of immunosuppressive therapy in HIV-negative patients [17].

The risk of developing PML-IRIS is related to the underlying predisposing factor for PML. Only 20% of HIV-infected patients with PML developed PML-IRIS [83], which contrasts with natalizumab-PML, where all patients (42) mostly treated with PLEX and IA developed PML-IRIS [143].

In the absence of clinical trials, there are no standard recommendations for the treatment of PML-IRIS, and treatment regimens are empirically driven [144]. Since PML-IRIS can be fatal and is associated with high disability, aggressive corticosteroid treatment has been advocated [129, 170, 171]. In a cohort of 54 HIV patients, 12 with PML-IRIS were treated with corticosteroids, of whom five died and seven showed a good neurological recovery. Patients who survived had received steroids early after PML-IRIS diagnosis and for longer durations, and had contrast enhancement on MRI [172]. In one case series of 42 natalizumab-related PML cases steroid use was associated with an improved outcome after IRIS [143]. The majority of published reports favour prompt corticosteroid use in PML-IRIS patients, but the dosage and duration of this treatment is not discussed.

Intravenous human immunoglobulin has been used in a few reported cases of PML-IRIS MS patients, with different outcomes: two patients significantly improved [113, 173], another survived [123] and one died of renal failure [123].

Maraviroc, an inhibitor of the CC-chemokine receptor 5 (CCR5), has recently emerged as an agent capable of preventing of PML-IRIS in some reports [174-176], but not in all [177]. CCR5 is expressed predominantly on T cells and macrophages, and less on B lineage cells, and it is involved in immune cell chemotaxis [178]. High numbers of CCR5 positive cells were found in PML-IRIS patients associated with HIV infection, natalizumab and immunosuppressive treatment [179]. Blockade of CCR5 might limit entry of CCR5 positive cells into the CNS, which might reduce the risk of IRIS-PML [174].

PROGNOSIS

In the past, PML diagnosed in the context of AIDS, lymphoproliferative diseases or immunosuppression invariably had a progressive course. Nowadays, although some patients still die within a few months, others experience disease stabilization and prolonged survival. The term progressive is thus no longer an accurate descriptor of PML. However, since remyelination does not occur in affected areas and there is high axonal damage, 80% of PML survivors are left with severe disability and quality of life may be poor [180].

In HIV-PML, survival has improved significantly, with a 1-year survival rate of about 46-58%, compared with 5% or lower in patients not receiving cART [72, 163, 181, 182]. The factors that appear to have a greater prognosis impact are a higher CD4+ count, low HIV RNA load, presence of JCV specific cytotoxic T lymphocytes, low JCV viral load in the CSF, inflammatory CSF profile, PML as the heralding manifestation of AIDS and older age [163]. The mortality due to natalizumab-PML has decreased over the years, with a survival rate greater than 70%, probably due to a combination of earlier detection and better understanding of how to manage the disease. In one study of natalizumab-PML, the survivors were younger, had lower pre-PML Expanded Disability Status Scale scores and a shorter time from symptom onset to diagnosis. Imaging features at diagnosis had a prognosis value, since 70% of those with fatal cases had widespread disease on brain MRI at diagnosis, while 86% of survivors had unilobar or multilobar disease

[171]. In another case series of natalizumab-PML, the mortality rate of PML-IRIS was approximately 25% [143].

Cases of asymptomatic PML identified on screening MRI have been associated with good clinical outcomes [183-185].

CONCLUSION

JCV is a common asymptomatic viral infection of humans, which in the setting of inadequate adaptive immune surveillance, causes the opportunistic infection PML.

Once a rare disease, PML has been considered an AIDS-defining illness since the HIV epidemic, and it has recently occurred as a consequence of effective therapies for autoimmune disease, such as natalizumab in MS patients. If in HIV patients PML management consists of in the optimization of cART, in MS patients on natalizumab treatment the most appropriate approach for PML is prevention, with careful selection of the appropriate therapy for each patient. If natalizumab is used in patients at high risk for PML, which is a course of action we do not recommend, constant vigilance is mandatory, as favourable outcomes are more likely if the disease is detected early.

ACKNOWLEDGMENT

We are grateful to Dr. Olinda Rebelo for the help with pathological studies.

REFERENCES

[1] Astrom K., Mancall E., Richardson E. P. Jr. (1958) Progressive multifocal leucoencephalopathy. *Brain,* 81:93-111.

[2] Richardson E. P. (1961) Progressive multifocal leukoencephalopathy. *N. Engl. J. Med.,* 1961, 265: 815-823.

[3] Cavanaugh J. B., Greenbaum D., Marshalll A., Rubinstein L. (1959) Cerebral demyelination associated with disorders of the reticuloendothelial system. *Lancet,* 524-529.

[4] Silverman L., Rubinstein L. J. (1965) Electron microscopic observations on a case of progressive multifocal leukoencephalopathy. *Acta. Neuropathol.*, 5: 215-224.

[5] Zu Rhein G. M., Chou S. M. (1965) Particles resembling papova viruses in human cerebral demyelinating disease. *Science,* 148: 1477-1479.

[6] Padgett B. L., Walker D. L., Zu Rhein G. M., Eckroade R. J. (1971) Cultivation of papova-like virus from human brain with progressive multifocal leukoencephalopathy. *Lancet,* 1:1257-1260.

[7] Miller J., Barret R., Britton C. (1982) Progressive multifocal leukoencephalopathy in a male homosexual with T-cell immune deficiency. *New Engl. J. Med.,* 307: 1436-1438.

[8] Holman R. C., Janssen R. S., Buehler J. W., Zelasky M. T., Hooper W. C. (1991) Epidemiology of progressive multifocal leukoencephalopathy in the United States: analysis of national mortality and AIDS surveillance data. *Neurology,* 41(11):1733-1736.

[9] Holman R. C., Török T. J., Belay E. D., Janssen R. S., Schonberger L. B. (1998) Progressive multifocal leukoencephalopathy in the United States, 1979-1994: increased mortality associated with HIV infection. *Neuroepidemiology*, 17(6):303-309.

[10] Casado J. L., Corral I., García J., Martinez-San Millán J., Navas E., Moreno A., Moreno S. (2014) Continued declining incidence and improved survival of progressive multifocal leukoencephalopathy in HIV/AIDS patients in the current era. *Eur. J. Clin. Microbiol. Infect. Dis.,* 33(2):179-87.

[11] Taoufik Y., Gasnault J., Karaterki A., Pierre Ferey M., Marchadier E., Goujard C. (1998) Prognostic value of JC virus load in cerebrospinal fluid of patients with progressive multifocal leukoencephalopathy. *J. Infect. Dis.,* 178(6):181620.

[12] Zheng H. C., Yan L., Cui L., Guan Y. F., Takanc Y. (2009) Mapping the history and current situation of research on John Cunningham virus a bibliometric analysis. *BMC Infect. Dis.,* 9:28.

[13] Focosi D., Marco T., Kast R. E., Maggi F., Ceccherini-Nelli L., Petrini M. (2010) Progressive multifocal leukoencephalopathy: what's new? *Neuroscientist,* 16(3):30823.

[14] Molloy E. S., Calabrese L. H. (2009) Progressive multifocal leukoencephalopathy: a national estimate of frequency in systemic lupus erythematosus and other rheumatic diseases. *Arthritis Rheum.,* 60(12):3761–5.

[15] Shitrit D., Lev N., Bar-Gil-Shitrit A., Kramer M. R. (2005) Progressive multifocal leukoencephalopathy in transplant recipients. *Transpl. Int.*, 17(11): 658-665.

[16] Calabrese L. H., Molloy E. S. (2008) Progressive multifocal leucoencephalopathy in the rheumatic diseases: assessing the risks of biological immunosuppressive therapies. *Ann. Rheum. Dis.*, 67(suppl. 3): iii64-iii65.

[17] Tan C. S., Koralnik I. J. (2010) Progressive multifocal leukoencephalopathy and other disorders caused by JC virus: clinical features and pathogenesis. *Lancet Neurol.*, 9:425–37.

[18] Jensen P. N., Major E. O. (2001) A classification scheme for human polyomavirus JCV variants based on the nucleotide sequence of the noncoding regulatory region. *J. Neurovirol.*, 7(4):280–7.

[19] Komagome R., Sawa H., Suzuki T., Suzuki Y., Tanaka S., Atwood W. J., et al. (2002) Oligosaccharides as receptors for JC virus. *J. Virol.*, 76(24):12992–3000.

[20] Gray J. A., Sheffler D. J., Bhatnagar A., Woods J. A., Hufeisen S. J., Benovic J. L., et al. (2001) Cell-type specific effects of endocytosis inhibitors on 5-hydroxytryptamine(2A) receptor desensitization and resensitization reveal an arrestin-, GRK2-, and GRK5-independent mode of regulation in human embryonic kidney 293 cells. *Mol. Pharmacol.*, 60(5):1020–30.

[21] Fonseca M. I., Ni Y. G., Dunning D. D., Miledi R. (2001) Distribution of serotonin 2A, 2C and 3 receptor mRNA in spinal cord and medulla oblongata. *Brain Res. Mol. Brain Res.*, 89(1-2):11–9.

[22] Cohen Z., Bouchelet I., Olivier A., Villemure J. G., Ball R., Stanimirovic D. B., et al. (1999) Multiple microvascular and astroglial 5-hydroxytryptamine receptor subtypes in human brain: molecular and pharmacologic characterization. *J. Cereb. Blood Flow Metab.*, 19(8): 908–17.

[23] Elphick G. F., Querbes W., Jordan J. A., Gee G. V., Eash S., Manley K., et al. (2004) The human polyomavirus, JCV, uses serotonin receptors to infect cells. *Science*, 306(5700):1380–3.

[24] Atwood W. J., Amemiya K., Traub R., Harms J., Major E. O. (1992) Interaction of the human polyomavirus, JCV, with human B-lymphocytes. *Virology*, 190(2):716–23.

[25] Monaco M. C., Jensen P. N., Hou J., Durham L. C., Major E. O. (1998) Detection of JC virus DNA in human tonsil tissue: evidence for site of initial viral infection. *J. Virol.*, 72(12):9918–23.

[26] Tan C. S., Dezube B. J., Bhargava P., Autissier P., Wuthrich C., Miller J., et al. (2009) Detection of JC virus DNA and proteins in the bone marrow of HIV-positive and HIV-negative patients: implications for viral latency and neurotropic transformation. *J. Infect. Dis.,* 199(6): 881-8.

[27] Adiele R. C., Adiele C. A. (2014) Progressive Multifocal Leukoencephalopathy. *J. Mult. Scler.,*1:2.

[28] Engels E. A., Rollison D. E., Hartge P., Baris D., Cerhan J. R., Severson R. K., et al. (2005) Antibodies to JC and BK viruses among persons with non-Hodgkin lymphoma. *Int. J. Cancer*, 117:1013–9.

[29] Olsson T., Achiron A., Alfredsson L., Berger T., Brassat D., Chan A., et al. (2013) Anti-JC virus antibody prevalence in a multinational multiple sclerosis cohort. *Mult. Scler.*, 19:1533–8.

[30] Bofill-Mas S., Girones R. (2003) Role of the environment in the transmission of JC virus. *J. Neurovirol.*, 9 Suppl. 1:54-8.

[31] Bofill-Mas S., Clemente-Casares P., Major E. O., Curfman B., Girones R. (2003) Analysis of the excreted JC virus strains and their potential oral transmission. *J. Neurovirol.,* 9(4):498-507.

[32] Berger J. R., Miller C. S., Mootoor Y., Avdiushko S. A., Kryscio R. J., Zhu H. (2006) JC virus detection in bodily fluids: clues to transmission. *Clin. Infect. Dis.,* 43(1):e9-12.

[33] Caldarelli-Stefano R., Vago L., Omodeo-Zorini E., Mediati M., Losciale L., Nebuloni M., et al. (1999) Detection and typing of JC virus in autopsy brains and extraneural organs of AIDS patients and non-immunocompromised individuals. *J. Neurovirol.*, 5(2):125-33.

[34] Monaco M. C., Atwood W. J., Gravell M., Tornatore C. S., Major E. O. (1996) JC virus infection of hematopoietic progenitor cells, primary B lymphocytes, and tonsillar stromal cells: implications for viral latency. *J. Virol.,* 70(10):7004–12.

[35] Randhawa P., Shapiro R., Vats A. (2005) Quantitation of DNA of polyomaviruses BK and JC in human kidneys. *J. Infect. Dis.,* 192(3): 504–9.

[36] Delbue S., Guerini F. R., Mancuso R., Caputo D., Mazziotti R., Saresella M., et al. (2007) JC virus viremia in interferon-beta-treated and untreated Italian multiple sclerosis patients and healthy controls. *J. Neurovirol.*, 13:73–7.

[37] Markowitz R. B., Thompson H. C., Mueller J. F., Cohen J. A., Dynan W. S. (1993) Incidence of BK virus and JC virus viruria in human

immunodeficiency virus-infected and -uninfected subjects. *J. Infect. Dis.*, 167(1):13–20.

[38] Kitamura T., Aso Y., Kuniyoshi N., Hara K., Yogo Y. (1990) High incidence of urinary JC virus excretion in nonimmunosuppressed older patients. *J. Infect. Dis.,* 161(6):1128–33.

[39] Ling P. D., Lednicky J. A., Keitel W. A., Poston D. G., White Z. S., Peng R., et al. (2003) The dynamics of herpesvirus and polyomavirus reactivation and shedding in healthy adults: a 14-month longitudinal study. *J. Infect. Dis*., 187:1571–80.

[40] Rossi A., Delbue S., Mazziotti R., Valli M., Borghi E., Mancuso R., et al. (2007) Presence, quantitation and characterization of JC virus in the urine of Italian immunocompetent subjects. *J. Med. Virol*., 79:408–12.

[41] Matos A., Duque V., Beato S., da Silva J. P., Major E., Meliço-Silvestre A. (2010) Characterization of JC human polyomavirus infection in a Portuguese population. *J. Med. Virol.,* 82:494–504.

[42] Yogo Y., Kitamura T., Sugimoto C., Ueki T., Aso Y., Hara K., et al. (1990) Isolation of a possible archetypal JC virus DNA sequence from nonimmunocompromised individuals. *J. Virol.,* 64(6):3139–43.

[43] Daniel A. M., Swenson J. J., Mayreddy R. P., Khalili K., Frisque R. J. (1996) Sequences within the early and late promoters of archetype JC virus restrict viral DNA replication and infectivity. *Virology*, 216:90–101.

[44] Van Loy T., Thys K., Ryschkewitsch C., Lagatie O., Monaco M. C., Major E. O., et al. (2015) JC Virus Quasispecies Analysis Reveals a Complex Viral Population Underlying Progressive Multifocal Leukoencephalopathy and Supports Viral Dissemination via the Hematogenous Route. *J. Virol.,* 89(2):1340-7.

[45] Wüthrich C., Kesari S., Kim W. K., Williams K., Gelman R., Elmeric D., et al. (2006) Characterization of lymphocytic infiltrates in progressive multifocal leukoencephalopathy: co-localization of CD8(+) T cells with JCV-infected glial cells. *J. Neurovirol*., 12(2):116-28.

[46] Khalili K., White M. K., Lublin F., Ferrante P., Berger J. R. (2007). Reactivation of JC virus and development of PML in patients with multiple sclerosis. *Neurology*, 68(13):985-90.

[47] Martin-Blondel G., Bauer J., Cuvinciuc V., Uro-Coste E., Debard A., Massip P., et al. (2013) In situ evidence of JC virus control by CD8+ T cells in PML-IRIS during HIV infection. *Neurology*, 81:964–70.

[48] Metz I., Radue E. W., Oterino A., Kumpfel T., Wiendl H., Schippling S., et al. (2012) Pathology of immune reconstitution inflammatory

syndrome in multiple sclerosis with natalizumab-associated progressive multifocal leukoencephalopathy. *Acta Neuropathol.*, 123:235–45.

[49] Koralnik I. J., Du Pasquier R. A., Letvin N. L. (2001) JC virus-specific cytotoxic T lymphocytes in individuals with progressive multifocal leukoencephalopathy. *J. Virol.*, 75:3483–7.

[50] Gheuens S., Bord E., Kesari S., Simpson D. M., Gandhi R. T., Clifford D. B. (2011) Role of CD4+ and CD8+ T-Cell Responses against JC Virus in the Outcome of Patients with Progressive Multifocal Leukoencephalopathy (PML) and PML with Immune Reconstitution Inflammatory Syndrome. *J. Virol.*, 85(14): 7256–7263.

[51] Plavina T., Subramanyam M., Bloomgren G., Richman S., Pace A., Lee S. (2014) Anti-JC virus antibody levels in serum or plasma further define risk of natalizumab-associated progressive multifocal leukoencephalopathy. *Ann. Neurol.*, 76(6):802-12.

[52] Shishido-Hara Y. (2010) Progressive multifocal leukoencephalopathy and promyelocytic leukemia nuclear bodies: a review of clinical, neuropathological, and virological aspects of JC virus-induced demyelinating disease. *Acta Neuropathol.*, 120(3):403-17.

[53] Kaplan J. E., Benson C., Holmes K. K., Brooks J. T., Pau A., Masur H. (2009) Guidelines for prevention and treatment of opportunistic infections in HIV-infected adults and adolescents: recommendations from CDC, the National Institutes of Health, and the HIV Medicine Association of the Infectious Diseases Society of America. *MMWR Recomm. Rep.*, 58(RR-4):1-207.

[54] Koralnik I. J., Wuthrich C., Dang X., Rottnek M., Gurtman A., Simpson D., et al. (2005) JC virus granule cell neuronopathy: A novel clinical syndrome distinct from progressive multifocal leukoencephalopathy. *Ann. Neurol.*, 57(4):576–80.

[55] Wuthrich C., Cheng Y. M., Joseph J. T., Kesari S., Beckwith C., Stopa E., et al. (2009) Frequent infection of cerebellar granule cell neurons by polyomavirus JC in progressive multifocal leukoencephalopathy. *J. Neuropathol. Exp. Neurol.*, 68(1):15–25.

[56] Wüthrich C., Dang X., Westmoreland S., McKay J., Maheshwari A., Anderson M. P., et al. (2009) Fulminant JC virus encephalopathy with productive infection of cortical pyramidal neurons. *Ann. Neurol.,* 65: 742–748.

[57] Gray F., Chretien F., Vallat-Decouvelaere A. V., Scaravilli F. (2003) The changing pattern of HIV neuropathology in the HAART era. *J. Neuropathol. Exp. Neurol.*, 62:429–440.

[58] Kuchelmeister K., Gullotta F., Bergmann M., Angeli G., Masini T. (1993) Progressive multifocal leukoencephalopathy (PML) in the acquired immunodeficiency syndrome (AIDS). A neuro-pathological autopsy study of 21 cases. *Pathol. Res. Pract.*, 189:163–173.

[59] Miralles P., Berenguer J., Lacruz C., Cosín J., López J. C., Padilla B., et al. (2001) Inflammatory reactions in progressive multifocal leukoencephalopathy after highly active antiretroviral therapy. *AIDS,* 15(14):1900-2.

[60] Safdar A., Rubocki R. J., Horvath J. A., Narayan K. K., Waldron R. L. (2002) Fatal immune restoration disease in human immunodeficiency virus type 1-infected patients with progressive multifocal leukoencephalopathy: impact of antiretroviral therapy-associated immune reconstitution. *Clin. Infect. Dis*., 35:1250–7.

[61] Hoffmann C., Horst H. A., Albrecht H., Schlote W. (2003) Progressive multifocal leucoencephalopathy with unusual inflammatory response during antiretroviral treatment. *J. Neurol. Neurosurg. Psychiatry,* 74: 1142–4.

[62] Di Giambenedetto S., Vago G., Pompucci A., Scoppettuolo G., Cingolani A., Marzocchetti A., et al. (2004) Fatal inflammatory AIDS-associated PML with high CD4 counts on HAART: a new clinical entity? *Neurology*, 63:2452–3.

[63] Vendrely A., Bienvenu B., Gasnault J., Thiebault J. B., Salmon D., Gray F. (2005) Fulminant inflammatory leukoencephalopathy associated with HAART-induced immune restoration in AIDS-related progressive multifocal leukoencephalopathy. *Acta Neuropathol.*, 109:449–455.

[64] Gray F., Bazille C., Adle-Biassette H., Mikol J., Moulignier A., Scaravilli F. (2005) Central nervous system immune reconstitution disease in acquired immunodeficiency syndrome patients receiving highly active antiretroviral treatment. *J. Neurovirol.*, 11(Suppl. 3): 16–22.

[65] Clifford D. B., Yiannoutsos C., Glicksman M., Simpson D. M., Singer E. J., Piliero P. J., et al. (1999) HAART improves prognosis in HIV-associated progressive multifocal leukoencephalopathy. *Neurology,* 52(3):623-5.

[66] Du Pasquier R. A., Koralnik I. J. (2003) Inflammatory reaction in progressive multifocal leukoencephalopathy: harmful or beneficial? *J. Neurovirol.*, 9(Suppl. 1):25–31.

[67] Cinque P., Bossolasco S., Brambilla A. M., Boschini A., Mussini C., Pierotti C., et al. (2003) The effect of highly active antiretroviral

therapy-induced immune reconstitution on development and outcome of progressive multifocal leukoencephalopathy: study of 43 cases with review of the literature. *J. Neurovirol.*, 9 Suppl. 1:73-80.

[68] Sadler M., Chinn R., Healy J., Fisher M., Nelson M. R., Gazzard B. G. (1998) New treatments for progressive multifocal leukoencephalopathy in HIV-1-infected patients. *Aids,* 12: 533–535.

[69] Kotecha N., George M. J., Smith T. W., Corvi F., Litofsky N. S. (1998) Enhancing progressive multifocal leukoencephalopathy: an indicator of improved immune status? *Am. J. Med.*, 105:541–543.

[70] Tantisiriwat W., Tebas P., Clifford D. B., Powderly W. G., Fichtenbaum C. J. (1999) Progressive multifocal leukoencephalopathy in patients with AIDS receiving highly active antiretroviral therapy. *Clin. Infect. Dis.*, 28:1152–1154.

[71] Collazos J., Mayo J., Martinez E., Blanco M. S. (1999) Contrastenhancing progressive multifocal leukoencephalopathy as an immune reconstitution event in AIDS patients. *AIDS*, 13:1426–1428.

[72] De Luca A., Giancola M. L., Ammassari A., Grisetti S., Paglia M. G., Gentile M., et al. (2000) The effect of potent antiretroviral therapy and JC virus load in cerebrospinal fluid on clinical outcome of patients with AIDS-associated progressive multifocal leukoencephalopathy. *J. Infect. Dis.*, 182(4):1077-83.

[73] Razonable R. R., Aksamit A. J., Wright A. J., Wilson J. W. (2001) Cidofovir treatment of progressive multifocal leukoencephalopathy in a patient receiving highly active antiretroviral therapy. *Mayo Clin. Proc.;* 76:1171–1175.

[74] Wyen C., Hoffmann C., Schmeisser N., Wöhrmann A., Qurishi N., Rockstroh J., et al. (2004) Progressive multifocal leukoencephalopathy in patients on highly active antiretroviral therapy: survival and risk factors of death. *J. Acquir. Immune Defic. Syndr.,* 37:1263–1268.

[75] Nuttall J. J., Wilmshurst J. M., Ndondo A. P., Yeats J., Corcoran C., Hussey G. D., Eley B. S. (2004) Progressive multifocal leukoencephalopathy after initiation of highly active antiretroviral therapy in a child with advanced human immunodeficiency virus infection: a case of immune reconstitution inflammatory syndrome. *Pediatr. Infect. Dis. J.,* 23:683–685.

[76] Kastrup O., Wanke I., Esser S., Maschke M. (2005) Evolution of purely infratentorial PML under HAART: negative outcome under rapid immune reconstitution. *Clin. Neurol. Neurosurg.*, 107:509–513.

[77] Wyen C., Lehmann C., Fatkenheuer G., Hoffmann C. (2005) AIDS-related progressive multifocal leukoencephalopathy in the era of HAART: report of two cases and review of the literature. *AIDS Patient Care STDS,* 19:486–494.

[78] Martinez J. V., Mazziotti J. V., Efron E. D., Bonardo P., Jordan R., Sevlever G., et al. (2006) Immune reconstitution inflammatory syndrome associated with PML in AIDS: a treatable disorder. *Neurology*, 67:1692–1694.

[79] Silva M. T., Pacheco M. C. Jr., Vaz B. (2006) Inflammatory progressive multifocal leukoencephalopathy after antiretroviral treatment. *Aids,* 20:469–471.

[80] D'Amico R., Sarkar S., Yusuff J., Azar E., Perlman D. C. (2007) Immune reconstitution after potent antiretroviral therapy in AIDS patients with progressive multifocal leukoencephalopathy. *Scand. J. Infect. Dis.*, 39:347–350.

[81] Lima M. A., Koralnik I. J. (2005) New features of progressive multifocal leukoencephalopathy in the era of highly active antiretroviral therapy and natalizumab. *J. Neurovirol.*, 11 suppl. 3:52–57.

[82] French M. A. (2009) HIV/AIDS: immune reconstitution inflammatory syndrome: a reappraisal. *Clin. Infect. Dis.*, 48: 101-107.

[83] Cinque P., Pierotti C., Vigano M. G., Bestetti A., Fausti C., Bertelli D., et al. (2001) The good and evil of HAART in HIV-related progressive multifocal leukoencephalopathy. *J. Neurovirol.,* 7:358–63.

[84] Langer-Gould A., Steinman L. (2005) Progressive multifocal leukoencephalopathy and multiple sclerosis: lessons from natalizumab. *Curr. Neurol. Neurosci. Rep.*, 6(3):253-8.

[85] Langer-Gould A., Atlas S. W., Green A. J., Bollen A. W., Pelletier D. (2005) Progressive multifocal leukoencephalopathy in a patient treated with natalizumab. *New Engl. J. Med.*, 353: 375-381.

[86] Van Assche G., Van Ranst M., Sciot R., Dubois B., Vermeire S., Noman M., et al. (2005) Progressive multifocal leukoencephalopathy after natalizumab therapy for Crohn's disease. *New Engl. J. Med.*, 362-368.

[87] Schmedt N., Andersohn F., Garbe E. (2012) Signals of progressive multifocal leukoencephalopathy for immunosuppressants: a disproportionality analysis of spontaneous reports within the US Adverse Event Reporting System (AERS). *Pharmacoepidemiol. Drug Saf.,* 21(11):1216-20.

[88] Wollebo H. S., White M. K., Gordon J., Berger J. R., Khalili K. (2015) Persistence and pathogenesis of the neurotropic polyomavirus JC. *Ann. Neurol.,* article in press.

[89] Stüve O., Gold R., Chan A., Mix E., Zettl U., Kieseier B. C. (2008) Alpha4-Integrin antagonism with natalizumab: effects and adverse effects. *J. Neurol.*, 255 Suppl. 6:58-65.

[90] Stüve O., Marra C. M., Bar-Or A., Niino M., Cravens P. D., Cepok S., et al. (2006) Altered CD4+/CD8+ T-cell ratios in cerebrospinal fluid of natalizumab-treated patients with multiple sclerosis. *Arch. Neurol.,* 63: 1383–7.

[91] Planas R., Jelcic I., Schippling S., Martin R., Sospedra M. (2012) Natalizumab treatment perturbs memory- and marginal zone-like B-cell homing in secondary lymphoid organs in multiple sclerosis. *Eur. J. Immunol.*, 42:790–8.

[92] Warnke C., Mausberg A. K., Stettner M., Dehmel T., Nekrich L., Meyer zu Horste G., et al. (2013) Natalizumab affects the T-cell receptor repertoire in patients with multiple sclerosis. *Neurology*, 81(16):1400-8.

[93] Hendel-Chavez H., de Goer de Herve M. G., Giannesini C., Mazet A. A., Papeix C., Louapre C., et al. (2013) Immunological hallmarks of JC virus replication in multiple sclerosis patients on long-term natalizumab therapy. *J. Virol.*, 87:6055–9.

[94] Chen Y., Bord E., Tompkins T., Miller J., Tan C. S., Kinkel R. P., et al. (2009) Asymptomatic reactivation of JC virus in patients treated with natalizumab. *N. Engl. J. Med.*, 361:1067–74.

[95] Bonig H., Wundes A., Chang K. H., Lucas S., Papayannopoulou T. (2008) Increased numbers of circulating hematopoietic stem/progenitor cells are chronically maintained in patients treated with the CD49d blocking antibody natalizumab. *Blood*, 111: 3439–3441.

[96] Zohren F., Toutzaris D., Klärner V., Hartung H. P., Kieseier B., Haas R. (2008) The monoclonal anti-VLA-4 antibody natalizumab mobilizes CD34+ hematopoietic progenitor cells in humans. *Blood,* 111: 3893–3895.

[97] Jing D., Oelschlaegel U., Ordemann R., Hölig K., Ehninger G., Reichmann H., et al. (2010) CD49d blockade by natalizumab in patients with multiple sclerosis affects steady-state hematopoiesis and mobilizes progenitors with a distinct phenotype and function. *Bone Marrow Transplant.*, 45: 1489–1496.

[98] Mattoscio M., Nicholas R., Sormani M. P., Malik O., Lee J. S., Waldman A. D., et al. (2015) Hematopoietic mobilization: Potential

biomarker of response to natalizumab in multiple sclerosis. *Neurology,* pii: 10.1212/WNL.0000000000001454.

[99] Frohman E. M., Monaco M. C., Remington G., Ryschkewitsch C., Jensen P. N., Johnson K., et al. (2014) C virus in CD341 and CD19+ cells in patients with multiple sclerosis treated with natalizumab. *JAMA Neurol.*, 71:596–602.

[100] Saure C., Warnke C., Zohren F., Schroeder T., Bruns I., Cadeddu R. P., et al. (2011) Natalizumab and impedance of the homing of CD34+ hematopoietic progenitors. *Arch. Neurol.*, 68:1428–1431.

[101] Warnke C., Smolianov V., Dehmel T., Andrée M., Hengel H., Zohren F., at al. (2010) CD34+ progenitor cells mobilized by natalizumab are not a relevant reservoir for JC virus. *Mult. Scler.*, 17:151–156.

[102] Carruthers R. L., Berger L. (2014) Progressive multifocal leukoencephalopathy and JC Virus-related disease in modern neurology practice. *Mult. Scler. Relat. Disord.*, 3, 419–430.

[103] Yousry T. A., Major E. O., Ryschkewitsch C., Fahle G., Fischer S., Hou J., et al. (2006) Evaluation of patients treated with natalizumab for progressive multifocal leukoencephalopathy. *N. Engl. J. Med.*, 354:924–933.

[104] Bloomgren G., Richman S., Hotermans C., Subramanyam M., Goelz S., Natarajan A., et al. (2012) Risk of natalizumab-associated progressive multifocal leukoencephalopathy. *N. Engl. J. Med.,* 366:1870–1880.

[105] Baldwin K. J., Hogg J. P. (2013) Progressive multifocal leukoencephalopathy in patients with multiple sclerosis. *Curr. Opin. Neurol.,* 26:318– 323.

[106] Sørensen P. S., Bertolotto A., Edan G., Giovannoni G., Gold R., Havrdova E., et al. (2012) Risk stratification for progressive multifocal leukoencephalopathy in patients treated with natalizumab. *Mult. Scler.,* 18(2):143-52.

[107] Schneider-Hohendorf T., Philipp K., Husstedt I. W., Wiendl H., Schwab N. (2014) Specific loss of cellular L-selectin on CD4(+) T cells is associated with progressive multifocal leukoencephalopathy development during HIV infection. *AIDS*, 28(5):793-5.

[108] Schwab N., Schneider-Hohendorf T., Posevitz V., Breuer J., Göbel K., Windhagen S., et al. (2013) L-selectin is a possible biomarker for individual PML risk in natalizumab-treated MS patients. *Neurology,* 81(10):865-71.

[109] Villar L. M., Costa-Frossard L., Masterman T., Fernandez O., Montalban X., Casanova B., et al. (2015) Lipid-Specific Immuno-

globulin M Bands in Cerebrospinal Fluid Are Associated with a Reduced Risk of Developing Progressive Multifocal Leukoencephalopathy during Treatment with Natalizumab. *Ann. Neurol.*, in press.

[110] Du Pasquier R. A., Pinschewer D. D., Merkler D. (2014) Immunological mechanism of action and clinical profile of disease-modifying treatments in multiple sclerosis. *CNS Drugs,* 28(6):535-58.

[111] Fine A. J., Sorbello A., Kortepeter C., Scarazzini L. (2014) Progressive multifocal leukoencephalopathy after natalizumab discontinuation. *Ann. Neurol.,* 75(1):108-15.

[112] Killestein J., Vennegoor A., van Golde A. E., Bourez R. L., Wijlens M. L., Wattjes M. P. (2014) PML-IRIS during Fingolimod Diagnosed after Natalizumab Discontinuation. *Case Rep. Neurol. Med.*, 307872.

[113] Calic Z., Cappelen-Smith C., Hodgkinson S. J., McDougall A., Cuganesan R., Brew B. J. (2015) Treatment of progressive multifocal leukoencephalopathy-immune reconstitution inflammatory syndrome with intravenous immunoglobulin in a patient with multiple sclerosis treated with fingolimod after discontinuation of natalizumab. *J. Clin. Neurosci.*, 22(3):598-600.

[114] http://www.novartis.com/newsroom/product-related-info-center/gilenya-safety.

[115] Bellizzi A., Anzivino E., Rodio D. M., Palamara A. T., Nencioni L., Pietropaolo V. (2013) New Insights on Human Polyomavirus JC and Pathogenesis of Progressive Multifocal Leukoencephalopathy. *Clin. Dev. Immunol.*, 2013:839719.

[116] Sahraian M. A., Radue E. W., Eshaghi A., Besliu S., Minagar A. (2012) Progressive multifocal leukoencephalopathy: a review of the neuroimaging features and differential diagnosis. *Eur. J. Neurol.,* 19(8):1060-9.

[117] Bernal-Cano F., Joseph J. T., Koralnik I. J. (2007) Spinal cord lesions of progressive multifocal leukoencephalopathy in an acquired immunodeficiency syndrome patient. *J. Neurovirol.*, 13:474–476.

[118] Kastrup O., Maschke M., Diener H. C., Wanke I. (2002) Progressive multifocal leukoencephalopathy limited to the brain stem. *Neuroradiology,* 44:227–229.

[119] Shintaku M., Matsumoto R., Sawa H., Nagashima K. (2000) Infection with JC virus and possible dysplastic ganglion-like transformation of the cerebral cortical neurons in a case of progressive multifocal leukoencephalopathy. *J. Neuropathol. Exp. Neurol.*, 59:921–929.

[120] Berger J. R., Kaszovitz B., Post M. J., Dickinson G. (1987) Progressive multifocal leukoencephalopathy associated with human immunodeficiency virus infection. A review of the literature with a report of sixteen cases. *Ann. Intern. Med.*, 107(1):78-87.
[121] Berger J. R. (2010) Progressive multifocal leukoencephalopathy and newer biological agents. *Drug Saf.*, 33(11):969-83.
[122] Lima M. A., Drislane F. W., Koralnik I. J. (2006) Seizures and their outcome in progressive multifocal leukoencephalopathy. *Neurology,* 66(2):262-4.
[123] Clifford D. B., De Luca A., Simpson D. M., Arendt G., Giovannoni G., Nath A. (2010) Natalizumab-associated progressive multifocal leukoencephalopathy in patients with multiple sclerosis: lessons from 28 cases. *Lancet Neurol.*, 9(4):438-46.
[124] Moreira I., Marta M. (2014) New and Old Concepts and Strategies for Progressive Multifocal Leukoencephalopathy. *J. Mult. Scler.*, 2:1.
[125] Hoepner R., Dahlhaus S., Kollar S., Zurawski B., Chan A., Kleiter I., et al. (2014) Prophylactic antiepileptic treatment reduces seizure frequency in natalizumab-associated progressive multifocal leukoencephalopathy. *Ther. Adv. Neurol. Disord.*, 7(1): 3–6.
[126] Berger J. R., Pall L., Lanska D., Whiteman M. (1998) Progressive multifocal leukoencephalopathy in patients with HIV infection. *J. Neurovirol.*, 4(1):59-68.
[127] Tortorella C., Direnzo V., D'Onghia M., Trojano M. (2013) Brainstem PML lesion mimicking MS plaque in a natalizumab-treated MS patient. *Neurology,* 81(16):1470-1.
[128] Berger J. R., Aksamit A. J., Clifford D. B., Davis L., Koralnik I. J., Sejvar J. J., et al. (2013) PML diagnostic criteria: consensus statement from the AAN Neuroinfectious Disease Section. Neurology, 80(15):1430-8.
[129] Wenning W., Haghikia A., Laubenberger J., Clifford D. B., Behrens P. F., Chan A., et al. (2009) Treatment of progressive multifocal leukoencephalopathy associated with natalizumab. *N. Engl. J. Med.,* 361:1075-1080.
[130] Calvi A., De Riz M., Pietroboni A. M., Ghezzi L., Maltese V., Arighi A., et al. (2014) Partial recovery after severe immune reconstitution inflammatory syndrome in a multiple sclerosis patient with progressive multifocal leukoencephalopathy. *Immunotherapy*, 6(1):23-8.
[131] Du Pasquier R. A., Corey S., Margolin D. H., Williams K., Pfister L. A., De Girolami U., et al. (2003) Productive infection of cerebellar granule

cell neurons by JC virus in an HIV+ individual. *Neurology*, 61(6): 775–82.

[132] Tyler K. L. (2003) The uninvited guest: JC virus infection of neurons in PML. *Neurology,* 61 (6):734–5.

[133] Behzad-Behbahani A., Klapper P. E., Vallely P. J., Cleator G. M., Bonington A. (2003) BKV-DNA and JCV-DNA in CSF of patients with suspected meningitis or encephalitis. *Infection,* 31(6):374– 8.

[134] Viallard J. F., Ellie E., Lazaro E., Lafon M. E., Pellegrin J. L. (2005) JC virus meningitis in a patient with systemic lupus erythematosus. *Lupus,* 14(12):964–6.

[135] Blake K., Pillay D., Knowles W., Brown D. W., Griffiths P. D., Taylor B. (1992) JC virus associated meningoencephalitis in an immunocompetent girl. *Arch. Dis. Child.*, 67(7):956–7.

[136] Yousry T. A., Pelletier D., Cadavid D., Gass A., Richert N. D., Radue E. W., et al. (2012) Magnetic resonance imaging pattern in natalizumab-associated progressive multifocal leukoencephalopathy. *Ann. Neurol.,* 72(5):779-87.

[137] Chang L., Ernst T., Tornatore C., Aronow H., Melchor R., Walot I., et al. (1997) Metabolite abnormalities in progressive multifocal leukoencephalopathy by proton magnetic resonance spectroscopy. *Neurology*, 48(4):836-45.

[138] Simone I. L., Federico F., Tortorella C., Andreula C. F., Zimatore G. B., Giannini P., et al. (1998) Localised 1H-MR spectroscopy for metabolic characterisation of diffuse and focal brain lesions in patients infected with HIV. *J. Neurol. Neurosurg. Psychiatry*, 64(4):516-23.

[139] Wattjes M. P., Richert N. D., Killestein J., de Vos M., Sanchez E., Snaebjornsson P., et al. (2013) The chameleon of neuroinflammation: magnetic resonance imaging characteristics of natalizumab-associated progressive multifocal leukoencephalopathy. *Mult. Scler.,* 19(14): 1826-40.

[140] Whiteman M. L., Post M. J., Berger J. R., Tate L. G., Bell M. D., Limonte L. P. (1993) Progressive multifocal leukoencephalopathy in 47 HIV-seropositive patients: neuroimaging with clinical and pathologic correlation. *Radiology,* 187(1):233-40.

[141] Khatri B. O. (2009) Therapeutic plasma exchange for worsening multiple sclerosis: does it work? *Expert Rev. Clin. Immunol.*, 5:491–493.

[142] Khatri B. O., Man S., Giovannoni G., Koo A. P., Lee J. C., Tucky B., et al. (2009) Effect of plasma exchange in accelerating natalizumab clearance and restoring leukocyte function. *Neurology,* 72(5):402-9.

[143] Tan I. L., McArthur J. C., Clifford D. B., Major E. O., Nath A. (2011) Immune reconstitution inflammatory syndrome in natalizumab-associated PML. *Neurology*, 77:1061–7.

[144] Dahlhaus S., Hoepner R., Chan A., Kleiter I., Adams O., Lukas C., et al. (2013) Disease course and outcome of 15 monocentrically treated natalizumab-associated progressive multifocal leukoencephalopathy patients. *J. Neurol. Neurosurg. Psychiatry*, 4(10):1068-74.

[145] Stüve O., Marra C. M., Cravens P. D., Singh M. P., Hu W., Lovett-Racke A., et al. (2007) Potential Risk of Progressive Multifocal Leukoencephalopathy With Natalizumab Therapy. *Arch. Neurol.,* 64(2): 169-76.

[146] Conomy J. P., Beard N. S., Matsumoto H., Roessmann U. (1974 Cytarabine treatment of progressive multifocal leukoencephalopathy. Clinical course and detection of virus-like particles after antiviral chemotherapy. *JAMA,* 229(10):1313-6.

[147] Hall C. D., Dafni U., Simpson D., Clifford D., Wetherill P. E., Cohen B., McArthur J., et al. (1998) Failure of cytarabine in progressive multifocal leukoencephalopathy associated with human immunodeficiency virus infection. AIDS Clinical Trials Group 243 Team. *N. Engl. J. Med.,* 338 (19): 1345-51.

[148] De Luca A., Ammassari A., Pezzotti P., Cinque P., Gasnault J., Berenguer J., et al. (2008) Cidofovir in addition to antiretroviral treatment is not effective for AIDS-associated progressive multifocal leukoencephalopathy: a multicohort analysis. *AIDS*, 22(14):1759-67.

[149] Royal W. 3rd, Dupont B., McGuire D., Chang L., Goodkin K., Ernst T., et al. (2003) Topotecan in the treatment of acquired immunodeficiency syndrome-related progressive multifocal leukoencephalopathy. *J. Neurovirol.*, 9(3):411-9.

[150] Huang S. S., Skolasky R. L., Dal Pan G. J., Royal W. 3rd, McArthur J. C. (1998) Survival prolongation in HIV-associated progressive multifocal leukoencephalopathy treated with alpha-interferon: an observational study. *J. Neurovirol.*, 4(3):324-32.

[151] Geschwind M. D., Skolasky R. I., Royal W. S., McArthur J. C. (2001) The relative contributions of HAART and alpha-interferon for therapy of progressive multifocal leukoencephalopathy in AIDS. *J. Neurovirol.,* 7(4):353-7.

[152] Nath A., Venkataramana A., Reich D. S., Cortese I., Major E. O. (2006) Progression of progressive multifocal leukoencephalopathy despite treatment with beta-interferon. *Neurology*, 66(1):149-50.

[153] Przepiorka D., Jaeckle K. A., Birdwell R. R., Fuller G. N., Kumar A. J., Huh Y. O., McCutcheon I. (1997) Successful treatment of progressive multifocal leukoencephalopathy with low-dose interleukin-2. *Bone Marrow Transplant.,* 20(11):983-7.

[154] Buckanovich R. J., Liu G., Stricker C., Luger S. M., Stadtmauer E. A., Schuster S. J., et al. (2002) Nonmyeloablative allogeneic stem cell transplantation for refractory Hodgkin's lymphoma complicated by interleukin-2 responsive progressive multifocal leukoencephalopathy. *Ann. Hematol.*, 81(7):410-3.

[155] Kunschner L., Scott T. F. (2005) Sustained recovery of progressive multifocal leukoencephalopathy after treatment with IL-2. *Neurology,* 65(9):1510.

[156] Abrams D., Lévy Y., Losso M. H., Babiker A., Collins G., Cooper D. A., et al. (2009) Interleukin-2 therapy in patients with HIV infection. *N. Engl. J. Med.*, 361(16):1548-59.

[157] Alstadhaug K. B., Croughs T., Henriksen S., Leboeuf C., Sereti I., Hirsch H. H., Rinaldo C. H. (2014) Treatment of progressive multifocal leukoencephalopathy with interleukin 7. *JAMA Neurol.,* 71(8):1030-5.

[158] Focosi D., Kast R. E., Maggi F., Ceccherini-Nelli L., Petrini M. (2007) Risperidone-induced reduction in JC viruria as a surrogate marker for efficacy against progressive multifocal leukoencephalopathy and hemorrhagic cystitis. *J. Clin. Virol.*, 39(1):63-4.

[159] Cettomai D., McArthur J. C. (2009) Mirtazapine use in human immunodeficiency virus-infected patients with progressive multifocal leukoencephalopathy. *Arch. Neurol.*, 66(2):255-258.

[160] Owczarczyk K., Hilker R., Brunn A., Hallek M., Rubbert A. (2007). Progressive multifocal leucoencephalopathy in a patient with sarcoidosis--successful treatment with cidofovir and mirtazapine. *Rheumatology (Oxford),* 46(5):888-90.

[161] Vulliemoz S., Lurati-Ruiz F., Borruat F. X., Delavelle J., Koralnik I. J., Kuntzer T., et al. (2006) Favourable outcome of progressive multifocal leucoencephalopathy in two patients with dermatomyositis. *J. Neurol. Neurosurg. Psychiatry,* 77(9):1079-1082.

[162] Kast R. E., Focosi D., Petrini M., Altschuler E. L. (2007) Treatment schedules for 5-HT2a blocking in progressive multifocal leukoencephalopathy using risperidone or ziprasidone. *Bone Marrow Transplant.*, 39(12):811-812.

[163] Marzocchetti A., Tompkins T., Clifford D. B., Gandhi R. T., Kesari S., Berger J. R., et al. (2009) Determinants of survival in progressive multifocal leukoencephalopathy. *Neurology*, 73:1551–8.
[164] Pöhlmann C., Hochauf K., Röllig C., Schetelig J., Wunderlich O., Bandt D. (2007) Chlorpromazine combined with cidofovir for treatment of a patient suffering from progressive multifocal leukoencephalopathy. *Intervirology,* 50(6):412-7.
[165] Brickelmaier M., Lugovskoy A., Kartikeyan R., Reviriego-Mendoza M. M., Allaire N., Simon K., et al. (2009) Identification and characterization of mefloquine efficacy against JC virus in vitro. *Antimicrob. Agents Chemother.*, 53(5):1840-1849.
[166] Schroder A., Lee D. H., Hellwig K., Lukas C., Linker R. A., Gold R. (2010) Successful management of natalizumab-associated progressive multifocal leukoencephalopathy and immune reconstitution syndrome in a patient with multiple sclerosis. *Arch. Neurol.,* 67(11):1391-4.
[167] McGuire J. L., Fridman V., Wuthrich C., Koralnik I. J., Jacobs D. (2011) Progressive multifocal leukoencephalopathy associated with isolated CD8+ T-lymphocyte deficiency mimicking tumefactive MS. *J. Neurovirol.,* 17(5):500-3.
[168] Kobayashi Z., Akaza M., Numasawa Y., Ishihara S., Tomimitsu H., Nakamichi K., et al. (2013) Failure of mefloquine therapy in progressive multifocal leukoencephalopathy: report of two Japanese patients without human immunodeficiency virus infection. *J. Neurol. Sci.*, 324(1-2): 190-4.
[169] Clifford D. B., Nath A., Cinque P., Brew B. J., Zivadinov R., Gorelik L., et al. (2013) A study of mefloquine treatment for progressive multifocal leukoencephalopathy: results and exploration of predictors of PML outcomes. *J. Neurovirol.*, 19(4): 351–358.
[170] Linda H., von Heijne A., Major E. O., Ryschkewitsch C., Berg J., Olsson T., et al. (2009) Progressive multifocal leukoencephalopathy after natalizumab monotherapy. *N. Engl. J. Med.*, 361(11):1081-7.
[171] Vermersch P., Kappos L., Gold R., Foley J. F., Olsson T., Cadavid D., et al. (2011) Clinical outcomes of natalizumab-associated progressive multifocal leukoencephalopathy. *Neurology,* 76(20):1697-704.
[172] Tan K., Roda R., Ostrow L., McArthur J., Nath A. (2009). PML-IRIS in patients with HIV infection. Clinical manifestations and treatment with steroids. *Neurology*, 72(17): 1458–1464.

[173] Kuhle J., Gosert R., Bühler R., Derfuss T., Sutter R., Yaldizli O., et al. (2011) Management and outcome of CSF-JC virus PCR- negative PML in a natalizumab-treated patient with MS. *Neurology*, 77(23):2010-6.

[174] Giacomini P. S., Rozenberg A., Metz I., Araujo D., Arbour N., Bar-Or A. and Group, Maraviroc in Multiple Sclerosis–Associated PML–IRIS (MIMSAPI) (2014) Maraviroc and JC Virus–Associated Immune Reconstitution Inflammatory Syndrome. *N. Engl. J. Med.*, 370(5):486-8.

[175] Martin-Blondel G., Cuzin L., Delobel P., Cuvinciuc V., Dumas H., Alvarez M., et al. (2009) Is maraviroc beneficial in paradoxical progressive multifocal leukoencephalopathy-immune reconstitution inflammatory syndrome management? *AIDS,* 23(18):2545-6.

[176] Ryerson L. Z. (2014) Maraviroc and JC - virus associated immune reconstitution inflammatory syndrome. ECTRIMS Online Library, 64558.

[177] Rodríguez M., Silva-Sánchez F. A., Luna-Rivero C., Vega-Barrientos R., Alvarado-de la Barrera C., Reyes-Terán G. (2014) Maraviroc Failed to Control Progressive Multifocal Leukoencephalopathy-Associated IRIS in a Patient with Advanced HIV Infection. *Case Reports in Medicine,* 2014:381480.

[178] Trebst C., Staugaitis S. M., Tucky B., Wei T., Suzuki K., Aldape K. D., et al. (2003) Chemokine receptors on infiltrating leucocytes in inflammatory pathologies of the central nervous system (CNS). *Neuropathol. Appl. Neurobiol.*, 29(6):584-95.

[179] Stork L., Brück W., Bar-Or A., Metz I. (2015) High CCR5 expression in natalizumab□associated progressive multifocal leukoencephalopathy immune reconstitution inflammatory syndrome supports treatment with the CCR5 inhibitor maraviroc. *Acta Neuropathol.*, 129(3):467-8.

[180] Koralnik I. J. (2006) Progressive multifocal leukoencephalopathy revisited: has the disease outgrown its name? *Ann. Neurol.*, 60:162–173.

[181] d'Arminio Monforte A., Cinque P., Mocroft A., Goebel F. D., Antunes F., Katlama C., et al. (2004) Changing incidence of central nervous system diseases in the EuroSIDA cohort. *Ann. Neurol.,* 55:320–8.

[182] Antinori A., Cingolani A., Lorenzini P., Giancola M. L., Uccella I., Bossolasco S., et al. (2003) Clinical epidemiology and survival of progressive multifocal leukoencephalopathy in the era of highly active antiretroviral therapy: data from the Italian Registry Investigative Neuro AIDS (IRINA). *J. Neurovirol.,* 9(Suppl. 1): S47–S53.

[183] Blair N. F., Brew B. J., Halpern J. P. (2012) Natalizumab-associated PML entified in the presymptomatic phase using MRI surveillance. *Neurology*, 78:507–8.

[184] Linda H., von Heijne A. (2013) Presymptomatic diagnosis with MRI and adequate treatment ameliorate the outcome after natalizumab- associated progressive multifocal leukoencephalopathy. *Front. Neurol.*, 4:11.

[185] Phan-Ba R., Lommers E., Tshibanda L., Calay P., Dubois B., Moonen G., et al. (2012) MRI preclinical detection and asymptomatic course of a progressive multifocal leucoencephalopathy (PML) under natalizumab therapy. *J. Neurol. Neurosurg. Psychiatry*, 83:224–6.

In: Progressive Multifocal Leukoencephalopathy ISBN: 978-1-63482-889-5
Editor: Denise S. Coleman

Chapter 2

Pathologic Features of Progressive Multifocal Leukoencephalopathy

Erika E. Doxtader, MD,*
and Richard A. Prayson, MD, MEd
Department of Pathology, Cleveland Clinic,
Cleveland, OH, US

Abstract

Progressive multifocal leukoencephalopathy (PML) is a rare demyelinating disease of the central nervous system caused by infection of oligodendrocytes by a papovavirus, most commonly JC virus. It typically occurs in immunocompromised individuals. This chapter focuses on the pathologic features of PML, characterized by a histologic triad of demyelination, intranuclear inclusions within oligodendrocytes, and enlarged reactive astrocytes with irregular, hyperchromatic nuclei. The demyelination most commonly occurs in subcortical regions of the brain and typically spares the spinal cord. The pathologic diagnosis can be confirmed by immunohistochemistry, in-situ hybridization, polymerase chain reaction or electron microscopy. We also discuss the differential diagnosis of the histologic findings, including other demyelinating diseases such as multiple sclerosis, acute disseminated

* Corresponding Author: Erika E. Doxtader, M.D. Department of Pathology, Cleveland Clinic Main Campus, Mail Code L25, 9500 Euclid Avenue, Cleveland, OH 44195, Tel: (216) 444-9154, Fax: (216) 445-6967, Email: doxtade@ccf.org.

encephalomyelitis/postvaccineal encephalomyelitis and acute necrotizing hemorrhagic leukoencephalitis.

Introduction

Progressive multifocal leukoencephalopathy (PML) is a demyelinating disorder of the central nervous system caused by opportunistic infection of oligodendrocytes by JC virus. It occurs almost exclusively in immunocompromised patients with impaired cell-mediated immunity. Åström and colleagues first described the pathologic features of PML in 1958 in a small autopsy series of patients who had underlying lymphoproliferative disorders [1]. Subsequent electron microscopic studies established a viral etiology, demonstrating the presence of polyoma-like virions within the nuclei of infected cells [2, 3].

The causative virus was later named JC virus, after John Cunningham, the patient in whom it was first isolated [4]. SV40 virus, another papovavirus, has also rarely been implicated [5]. BK virus has not been implicated in the pathogenesis of PML.

Today, PML is most commonly seen in patients with human immunodeficiency virus/acquired immunodeficiency syndrome (HIV/AIDS), and has also been reported in individuals treated with monoclonal antibodies such as natalizumab (used for the treatment of multiple sclerosis and Crohn's disease) and rituximab (used to treat B-cell lymphomas and some autoimmune diseases) [6, 7, 8].

Definitive diagnosis of PML requires demonstration of JC virus within the central nervous system in the appropriate clinical and radiologic context [9]. In many cases, the presence of JC virus can be demonstrated by polymerase chain reaction (PCR) of cerebrospinal fluid (CSF). However, in cases where clinical or radiological features are atypical, or when CSF PCR for JC virus is negative, the diagnosis may require stereotactic brain biopsy [9, 10].

This chapter focuses on the macroscopic and microscopic pathologic features of PML and discusses ancillary studies that are helpful for identifying the virus within infected tissue. The pathologic differential diagnosis is also reviewed, with emphasis on pitfalls and histologic features useful in the differential diagnosis. Limitations related to tissue sampling are also discussed.

Clinical Features

Patients with PML often present with focal neurologic deficits, such as limb weakness, visual loss, and cognitive abnormalities. Patients with cerebellar involvement may have ataxia.

Radiographic Features

Computed tomography (CT) typically shows hypodense white matter lesions. T2-weighted magnetic resonance imaging (MRI) shows multifocal hyperintense white matter signal abnormalities. Enhancement and mass effect are generally not present. MRI is more sensitive than CT scan for detecting lesions of PML [11]. Lesions preferentially are located in the subcortical white matter.

Macroscopic Features

The gross features of PML are only appreciated at autopsy. The demyelinating lesions manifest as multiple, usually bilateral tiny grey or brown areas of discoloration located predominantly in the subcortical white matter at the grey matter-white matter junction [1, 12]. The lesions are most frequent in the cerebral hemispheres, and have a predilection for the parietal and occipital lobes (Figure 1).

A study of 47 cases with radiologic-pathologic correlation documented demyelinating foci of PML in the subcortical white matter, periventricular white matter, corpus callosum, internal capsule, small myelinated fibers of the thalamus and basal ganglia, and posterior fossa. The majority of patients (79%) had bilateral lesions [11]. The spinal cord and optic nerve are almost always uninvolved [12]. The demyelinating foci range from 1-2 millimeters to large destructive lesions measuring several centimeters in diameter. Large lesions result from coalescence of smaller lesions, and may become cavitated [1, 6, 12].

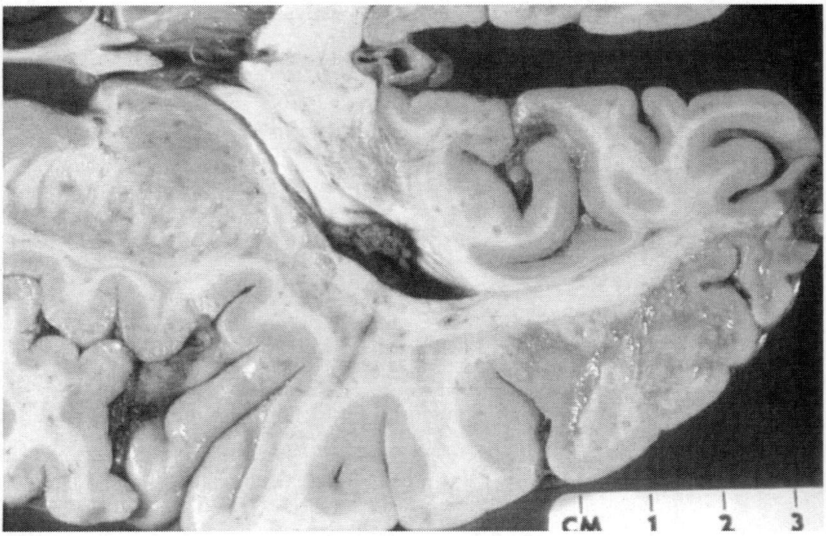

Figure 1. Gross appearance of progressive multifocal leukoencephalopathy. A confluent zone of subcortical demyelination is present in the occipital lobe.

MICROSCOPIC FEATURES

The histologic triad of PML consists of:

1. Demyelination. The predominant microscopic finding in PML is active demyelination, characterized on routine hematoxylin and eosin (H&E) -stained sections by sheets of macrophages with abundant foamy cytoplasm (Figure 2). Macrophages can be highlighted using antibody immunostaining (e.g. CD68). Other inflammatory cells are usually absent, although a few lymphocytes (typically benign appearing T lymphocytes) may be present around blood vessels [1, 3, 12]. Loss of myelin can be highlighted with a myelin stain such as Luxol fast blue, which shows areas of loss of blue-staining myelin within the neuropil, and accumulation of myelin-rich debris within macrophages (Figure 3). Axons remain relatively preserved; they can be demonstrated with immunohistochemistry for neurofilament protein.
2. Oligodendrocytes with enlarged, round nuclei containing viral inclusions. These cells are present in variable numbers within the

inflammatory infiltrate (Figure 4), and usually predominate at the edge of the lesion [11, 12]. The nuclei are approximately 2-3 times the size of a normal oligodendrocyte nucleus. The viral inclusions typically occupy most of the nucleus, displacing internal nuclear structures like chromatin; these inclusions are sometimes referred to as Cowdry type A inclusions. This is in contrast to the smaller intranuclear Cowdry B inclusions that do not displace internal nuclear structures. The viral inclusions in PML usually appear purple, homogeneous and glassy. However, they may also appear dark and smudgy (Figure 5), or well defined and eosinophilic, surrounded by a zone of chromatin clearing and with a well-defined rim of marginated chromatin (Figure 6).

3. Bizarre astrocytes. Reactive astrocytes with abundant dense eosinophilic cytoplasm, peripherally located nuclei, and radiating cell processes are often present. Bizarre astrocytic cells with pleomorphic, enlarged multilobated nuclei may also be seen, although their presence is variable from case to case [12] (Figure 7). These atypical astrocytes have been sometimes referred to as Alzheimer type I astrocytes. Mitotic figures, including atypical forms, may be present (Figure 8).

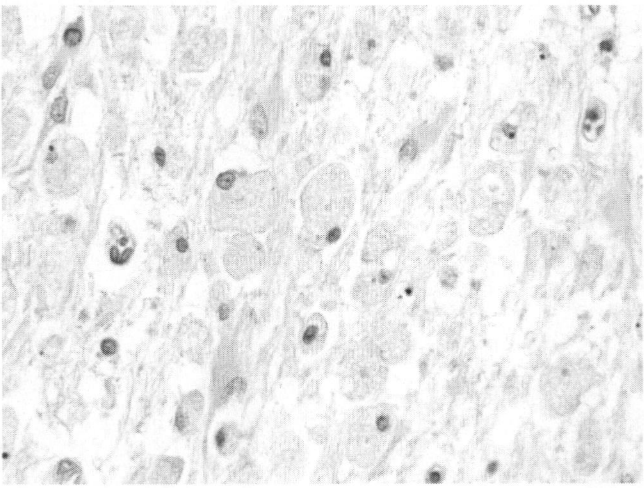

Figure 2. Macrophage infiltrate in progressive multifocal leukoencephalopathy. The macrophages have abundant, pale pink, foamy cytoplasm and well-defined cell borders. A few reactive astrocytes are also present (H&E, original magnification, 400x).

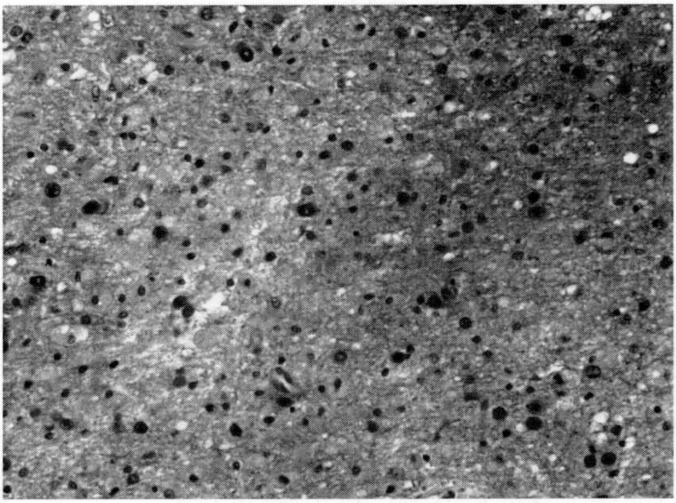

Figure 3. Demyelination in progressive multifocal leukoencephalopathy. An area of myelin loss appears pale pink (left), in contrast to the blue staining of the myelinated tissue at the right (Luxol fast blue, original magnification, 200x).

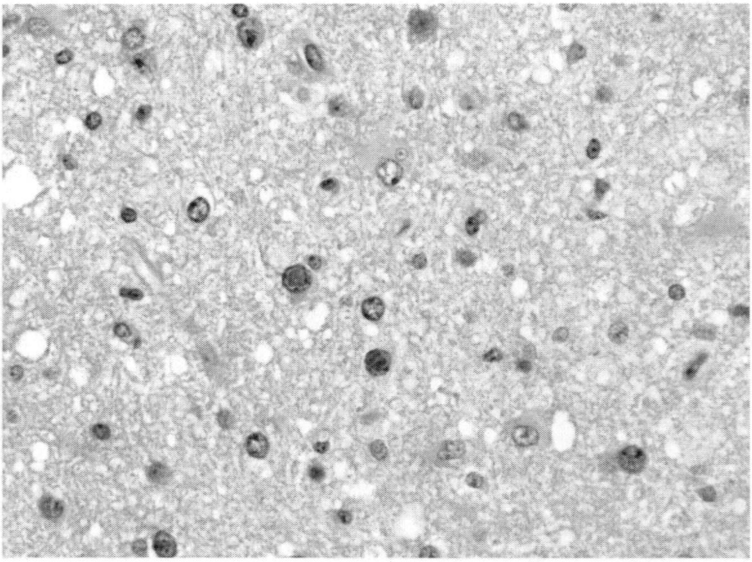

Figure 4. Abnormal oligodendrocyte nuclei in progressive multifocal leukoencephalopathy. Glassy, purple viral inclusions are numerous (H&E, original magnification, 400x).

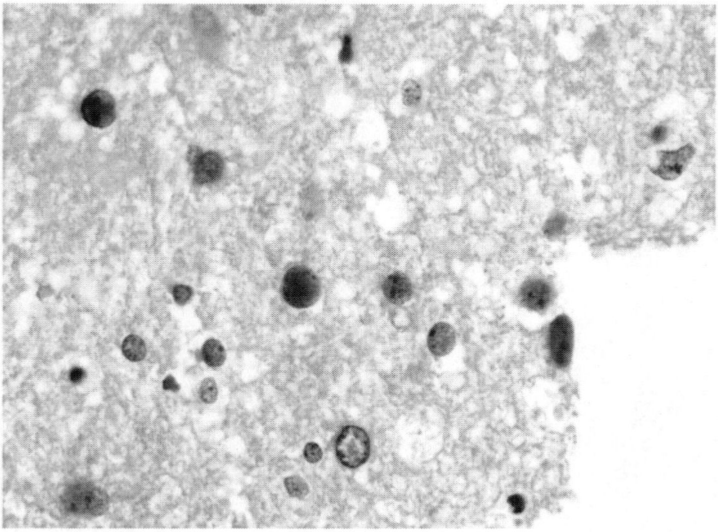

Figure 5. Viral inclusion in progressive multifocal leukoencephalopathy. An enlarged oligodendrocyte nucleus has the characteristic homogenous, smudgy dark purple appearance (H&E, original magnification, 600x).

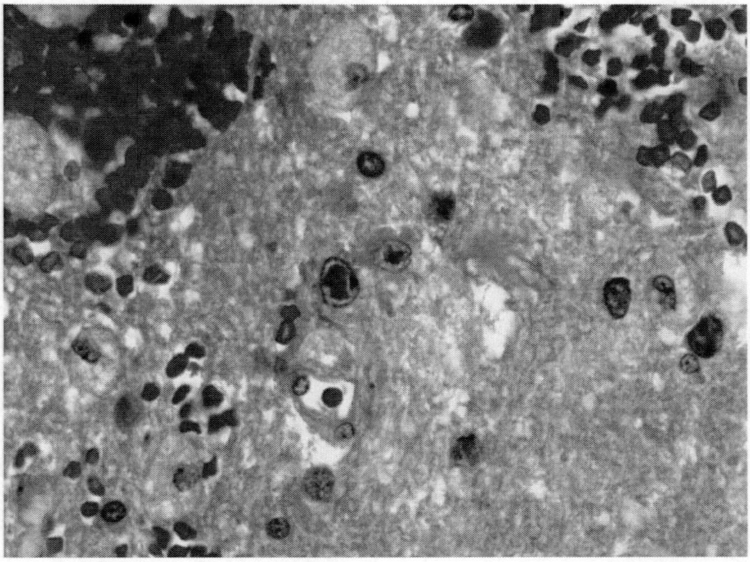

Figure 6. Oligodendrocyte nucleus in a case of progressive multifocal leukoencephalopathy. This viral inclusion is well defined and surrounded by nuclear clearing and marginated chromatin (H&E, original magnification, 600x).

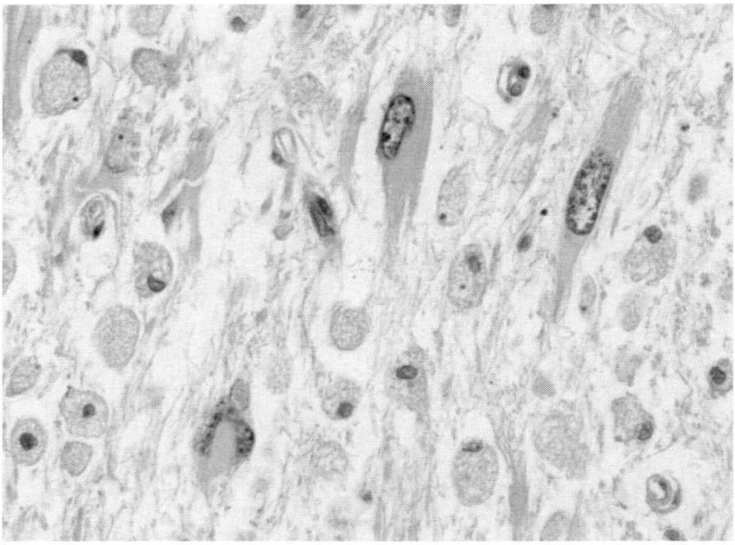

Figure 7. Bizarre astrocytes with enlarged, atypical nuclei in progressive multifocal leukoencephalopathy. The nuclei are elongated and have a glassy appearance with clumped chromatin. A multilobated form is present (H&E, original magnification 400x).

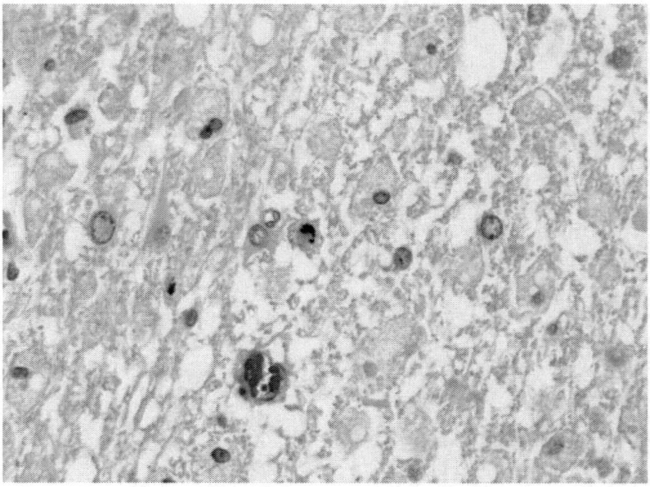

Figure 8. A mitotic figure is present in this example of progressive multifocal leukoencephalopathy. Mitoses may raise the differential diagnostic consideration of astrocytoma, especially when bizarre astrocytes are present (H&E, original magnification, 400x).

The pathologic diagnosis can be made on small biopsies, provided that diagnostic infected oligodendrocytes are present. Since the distribution of these cells is not uniform throughout the lesion, and they are often located peripherally, tissue sampling may become an issue. Management of tissue and determination of specimen adequacy at the time of frozen section is essential to ensure that diagnostic material is obtained [10]. If demyelination is suspected at the time of frozen section, tissue can be fixed in glutaraldehyde for electron microscopic (EM) examination. Additional tissue should be requested if diagnostic infected oligodendroglial cells are not seen at the time of frozen section, and clinical suspicion is high.

ANCILLARY STUDIES

Many ancillary techniques are available to demonstrate JC virus within lesional brain tissue, including immunohistochemistry, in-situ hybridization, PCR, and electron microscopy. Immunohistochemical staining for JC virus or SV40 (a related papovavirus) is the easiest. It allows visual confirmation of viral antigens within infected oligodendrocyte nuclei and astrocyte nuclei (Figure 9). In-situ hybridization and PCR, including pyrosequencing, may also be used to demonstrate the presence of viral DNA in paraffin-embedded tissue [6, 13, 14]. Electron microscopy reveals filamentous and spherical viral particles measuring approximately 40 mμ in diameter within oligodendrocyte nuclei (Figure 10) [2, 3].

DIFFERENTIAL DIAGNOSIS

The pathologic differential diagnosis includes astrocytoma, other demyelinating diseases, other infections, and infarct.

Astrocytic neoplasms enter the differential diagnosis due to the hypercellularity of the lesions of PML, especially if atypical astrocytic cells and mitotic figures are present. At frozen section, the irregularly shaped nuclei of macrophages may be misconstrued as malignant astrocytes, if the cytoplasmic features of the cells are not clearly discernible. The atypia encountered in the Alzheimer type I astrocytes can look very similar to the atypia encountered in a malignancy; the tip-off to the correct diagnosis is the presence of macrophages, which are common in PML and rare in astrocytic tumors (unless they have been previously radiated). The presence of white matter macrophages should prompt the pathologist to consider a demyelinating lesion rather than a neoplasm [15]. Recognition of viral inclusions within oligodendrocytes is essential to arrive at the correct diagnosis. Isocitrate dehydrogenase 1 (IDH-1) antibody can be useful in this differential diagnosis as well, since many (but not all) World Health Organization grade II gliomas are positive and PML would be negative [16].

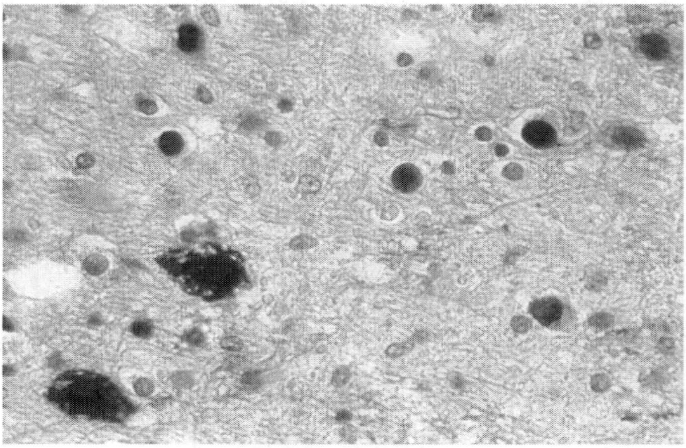

Figure 9. Immunohistochemical stain for JC virus in progressive multifocal leukoencephalopathy. Both oligodendrocytes and astrocytes stain positively (JC immunostain, original magnification, 400x).

Other demyelinating diseases also enter the differential diagnosis. Acute or subacute multiple sclerosis may histologically resemble PML in that lesions, also referred to as plaques, may feature sharply demarcated foci of active demyelination, but viral inclusions are absent. Most plaques are classically periventricular in location. Spinal cord and optic nerve involvement by multiple sclerosis are relatively common in contrast to PML. Alzheimer type I astrocytes are generally not encountered in multiple sclerosis.

Acute disseminated encephalomyelitis (ADEM), another demyelinating disorder, is seen primarily in children and is often preceded by a viral infection or prior vaccination. The pattern of demyelination in this disorder is characteristically perivenular. Acute hemorrhagic leukoencephalitis, a more fulminant form of ADEM, features perivenular demyelination, fibrinoid necrosis of vessel walls, and perivascular hemorrhages. Diagnostic features of

PML such as intranuclear Cowdry A inclusions and Alzheimer type I astrocytes are not present in these two disorders [17].

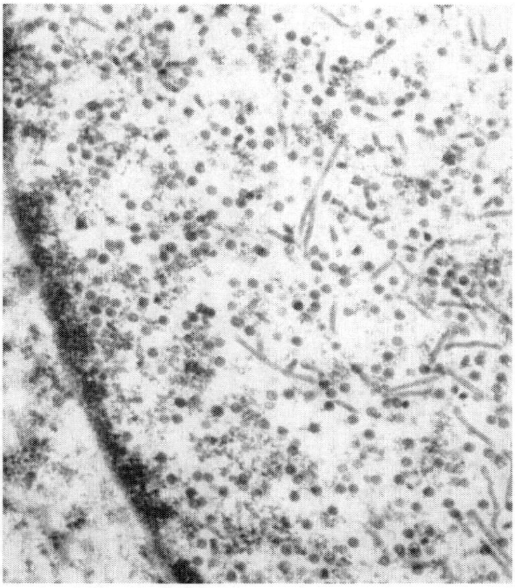

Figure 10. Ultrastructural findings in progressive multifocal leukoencephalopathy. Spherical and filamentous viral particles are present within an oligodendrocyte nucleus.

Subacute sclerosing panencephalitis, a rare disorder seen in children that is caused by a defective measles virus, may also contain intranuclear inclusions within oligodendrocytes that appear similar to those of PML. Demyelination is not a feature, however [17]. Other infections that feature macrophages also enter the differential diagnosis, especially in the setting of a patient with HIV/AIDS. Toxoplasmosis is characterized by necrosis and a mixed inflammatory infiltrate composed of macrophages, lymphocytes, and neutrophils. In contrast, the infiltrate in PML is characteristically macrophage-rich, and does not typically contain many other inflammatory cells. *Toxoplasma* cysts containing numerous bradyzoites can establish the correct diagnosis. Numerous macrophages are also seen in disseminated histoplasmosis, but yeast forms are readily visible within macrophages on H&E or with Gomori methenamine silver staining in this condition. Rare cases of *Mycobacterium avium* complex may be marked by prominent numbers of macrophages that are filled with acid-fast organisms. Most of these other infectious diseases also involve grey matter, which would not be the case in PML.

A subacute or chronic infarct may also mimic demyelination histologically, in that numerous macrophages and reactive astrocytes may be present. However, infarcts feature loss of both myelin and axons, whereas demyelinating lesions show loss of myelin but preservation of axons. Myelin stains such as Luxol fast blue and immunohistochemistry for neurofilament can be helpful in making this distinction. Reactive astrocytes in an infarct are situated around the perimeter of the lesion in contrast to demyelinating disorders where reactive astrocytes are situated within the zones of demyelination.

CONCLUSION

Pathologists should recognize the pathologic features of PML, since the diagnosis is occasionally based on histologic findings. The histologic triad of demyelination, enlarged oligodendrocyte nuclei containing viral inclusions, and bizarre astrocytes is characteristic. Demonstration of JC virus within affected tissue is diagnostic.

REFERENCES

[1] Åström KE, Mancall EL, Richardson EP, Jr. Progressive multifocal leuko-encephalopathy. A hitherto unrecognized complication of chronic lymphatic leukemia and Hodgkin's disease. *Brain* 1958;81:93-111.

[2] Howatson AF, Nagai M, and ZU Rhein GM. Polyoma-like virions in human demyelinating brain disease. *Canad. Med. Ass. J.* 1965;93:379-86.

[3] Dolman CL, Furesz J, Mackay B. Progressive multifocal leukoencephalopathy: Two cases with electron microscopic and viral studies. *Canad. Med. Ass. J.* 1967;97:8-12.

[4] Padgett BL, Walker DL, ZuRhein GM, Eckroade RJ. Cultivation of papova-like virus from human brain with progressive multifocal leukoencephalopathy. *Lancet* 1971;1:1257-60.

[5] Weiner LP, Herndon RM, Narayan O, *et al.* Isolation of virus related to SV40 from patients with progressive multifocal leukoencephalopathy. *N. Eng. J. Med.* 1972;286:385-390.
[6] Kleinschmidt-DeMasters BK and Tyler KL. Progressive multifocal leukoencephalopathy complicating treatment with natalizumab and interferon beta-1a for multiple sclerosis. *N. Eng. J. Med.* 2005;353:369-74.
[7] Bloomgren G, Richman S, Hotermans C, *et al.* Risk of natalizumab-associated progressive multifocal leukoencephalopathy. *N. Eng. J. Med.* 2012;366:1870-80.
[8] Carson KR, Evens AM, Richey EA, *et al.* Progressive multifocal leukoencephalopathy after rituximab therapy in HIV-negative patients: a report of 57 cases from the Research on Adverse Drug Events and Reports Project. *Blood* 2009;113:4834-40.
[9] Burger JR, Aksamit AJ, Clifford DB, *et al.* PML diagnostic criteria. Consensus statement from the AAN neuroinfectious disease section. *Neurology* 2013;80:1430-8.
[10] Prayson RA, Estes ML. Stereotactic brain bicpsy for diagnosis of progressive multifocal leukoencephalopathy. *South Med. J.* 1993;86:1381-4, 1394.
[11] Hansman Whiteman ML, Donovan Post MJ, Berger JR, *et al.* Progressive multifocal leukoencephalopathy in 47 HIV-seropositive patients: neuroimaging with clinical and pathologic correlation. *Radiology* 1993;187:233-40.
[12] Richardson EP, Jr. Progressive multifocal leukoencephalopathy. *N. Eng. J. Med.* 1961;265:815-23.
[13] Arthur RR, Dagostin S, Shah KV. Detection of BK virus and JC virus in urine and brain tissue by the polymerase chain reaction. *J. Clin. Microbiol.* 1989;27:1174-9.
[14] Telenti A, Aksamit Jr. AJ, Proper J, and Smith TF. Detection of JC virus DNA by polymerase chain reaction in patients with progressive multifocal leukoencephalopathy. *J. Infect. Dis.* 1990;162:858-61.
[15] Love S. Demyelinating diseases. *J Clin Pathol* 2006;59:1151-9.
[16] Capper D, Sahm F, Hartmann C, *et al.* Application of mutant IDH1 antibody to differentiate diffuse glioma from nonneoplastic central nervous system lesions and therapy-induced changes. *Am. J. Surg. Pathol.* 2010;34:1199-1204.
[17] Prayson RA. Neuropathology: A volume in the series Foundations in diagnostic pathology. 2nd ed. Philadelphia, PA: Saunders;2012.

In: Progressive Multifocal Leukoencephalopathy ISBN: 978-1-63482-889-5
Editor: Denise S. Coleman

Chapter 3

RISK FACTORS AND TREATMENT OF PROGRESSIVE MULTIFOCAL LEUKOENCEPHALOPATHY

David Pérez-Callejo*[*], *Isabel Curto and Mariano Provencio

Medical Oncology Department, Hospital Universitario Puerta de Hierro Majadahonda, Madrid, Spain

ABSTRACT

Progressive multifocal leukoencephalopathy (PML) is a neurological potencially fatal disease caused by JC polyomavirus, most often seen among patients with severe defects in the cellular immune system. Despite an 80% estimated seroprevalence of anti-JC virus antibodies in healthy people, development of symptoms in non-immunocompromised individuals is extremely rare.

Historically, this disease have gone through three big periods: in the early 1980s, PML was initially described in patients with lymphoproliferative diseases; with the acquired immune deficiency syndrome (AIDS) pandemic, PML affected 4-5% of all human immunodeficiency virus (HIV)-infected patients. Nowadays, after the development of antiretroviral therapy, and with the use of several monoclonal antibodies for cancer and autoimmune diseases, specially

[*] Email: davidperezc@hotmail.com.

natalizumab-related multiple sclerosis, psoriasis treatment with efalizumab, and the widely use of rituximab, several cases have started to be more frequently described in these patients treated with these immunosupressants.

Typically, this infection will affect olygodendrocytes and their myelin processes, and symptoms will vary depending on the areas of demyelination. Its diagnosis will be confirmed after detection of viral DNA or proteins by in situ hybridation or by immunohistochemistry on a brain biopsy or after JC virus detection by a positive polymerase chain reaction (PCR) in the cerebrospinal fluid (CSF).

No treatment provided demonstrable therapeutic efficacy. Several clinical cases and small trials have been reported with different drugs including antineoplastic, immunomodulants, antiviral and antimalarial agents or serotoninergic antagonists; with many of the affected individuals dying from this disease. Because of all these failed efforts, immune reconstitution syndrome remains to be the most important and effective approach to treatment, with antiretrovirals as the standard therapy for HIV-patients and with worse outcome for non-HIV patients, since it is not always possible to withdraw their immunosupresive medication because of the risk.

Because PML still has today a high mortality rate, a development of treatments are urgently needed to impact in the survival of these individuals.

INTRODUCTION

Progressive multifocal leukoencephalopathy (PML) is a rare, opportunistic and demiyelinating infection of the central nervous system (CNS) caused by John Cunningham (JC) virus [1]. It mainly occurs in patients with severe cellular immunosupression. Since HIV pandemic, AIDS has become the principal risk factor [2].

Most cases reported occur in HIV-infected patients (80%), patients with hematological malignancies (13%) and transplant recipients with immunosuppressant medication (5%). Moreover, it has been described also in autoinmmune disorders and chronic inflammatory joint diseases (2%) [3].

Since the development of several monoclonal antibodies (mAb), PML-related cases have also been described.

There has been no discovery of effective antiviral curative therapy against this virus. To date, several treatments for PML has been evaluated for effectiveness, but favourable outcomes have not been reported yet [4, 5].

JC VIRUS

JC virus belongs to the subgroup of *polyomaviridae* of the family *Papovaviridae* [6]. Other viruses of this family are BK virus, simian vacuolating virus (SV40), KI virus, WU virus and Merkel cell virus [1].

JC virus is a small ubiquitous DNA polyomavirus with 5.13 kb circular enclosed double-stranded DNA [1, 7]. The JC virus genome is organized in different functional regions: the coding and the non-coding region.

The coding region, which comprises about 90% of the viral genome, confers the genotype that is associated with the different types found. In this region remain the early genes and the late genes [7, 8].

The early genes encoded the large T regulatory protein which is a DNA binding protein, necessary for replication and transcription and the small t antigen that participate in viral multiplication and is related to pathogenicity in humans [7, 8]. The late genes encode: the capsid protein VP1, which is the responsible of icosahedral structure and contains epitopes for antibody induction and recognitio; VP2 and VP3 which have a role in propagation; and agnoprotein, acting like a viroporin that can downregulate T protein activity [1, 7] The coding region has not been associated with pathogenesis.

The regulatory region is a non-coding region that contains the origin of replication, viral promoter-enhancing sequences and binding sites for cell transcription factors. It is hypervariable and have rearrangements; it is known as the " archetype" and contains determinants for neurotropism and neurovirulence. These rearranged regions most likely form during immunosupression and are necessary for JC virus reactivation. Their detection in plasma is related to poor clinical outcome. Moreover, replication and transcription depend on binding of nuclear factors to specific sites in the regulatory region. The viral transcription is proportional to number of binding sites [7].

In initial adhesion of JC virus to cells that get infected, N-linked glycoprotein with alpha 2,3- or alpha 2,8 linked sialic acids are involved. Subsequently, specific interaction with serotonin receptor is taken place. An endocytosis takes place and finally DNA is transferred to the nucleus. Then, early gene expression is taken place, followed by genome replication and late gene expression. Finally, the virus is assembled [1].

JC virus is distributed worldwide and antibodies against JC virus are detected in over 80% world population [1]. The haemagglutination inhibiton assay detected a seroprevalence of 60% in individuals aged 20-29 years in the USA. Other assays have detected a seroprevalence of 50% in individuals aged

60-69 years in Wales and England or about 80% in Germany. It is reported that in other US study the seroprevalence was 39% and 65 %, respectively for a similar category groups [7].

It has been suggested JC virus to play a possible role in several types of cancer [1].

PROGRESSIVE MULTIFOCAL LEUKOENCEFALOPATHY

PML was initially described in three patients with hematological malignancies in 1958 by Astrom *et al.* [1, 9]. The viral nature of PML was first postulated in 1959 and then confirmed by Zu Rhein and co-workers in 1967, observing polyoma-like virions on electron microscopy of a tissue sample from a patient with PML. It was named JC virus by Padgett and colleagues based on the initials of the patient from who it was first isolated in 1971 [10].

After an asymptomatic primary infection in the childhood, the virus remains latent [7].

The mechanism of viral transmission remains controversial, although inhalation and ingestion of contaminated water or food have been proposed as major modes of transmission between people [8, 10].

The JC virus has tropism for different tissues. It was isolated from tonsilar stromal cells and B-cell lymphocytes. It is thought that it is spread via respiratory inhalation and tonsils serving as potential sites for initial infection. Peripheral blood cells are possible reservoirs. Bone narrow and kidney are sites of latent infection with JC virus being also excreted in urine of patients with PML and healthy humans [1]. CNS has been suggested as a possible site of persistence too [8].

The way virus JC infects CNS is still not completely understood, with two possibilities suggested and not exlusive: either the virus only infects CNS after reactivation in other places of the body where it is latent, in the context of an alteration of immune response or the virus is infecting CNS remaining there for many years controlled by T-cells, and it emerges when there is an alteration in the immune system [1].

On the other hand, increased levels of specific antibodies against JC virus not prevent the onset of the disease. CD4-CD8 cell-mediated immunity has an important role in the anti JCV immune reponse. Recognition of antigens presented by MHC-class II by CD4+cells and subsequent cytotoxic CD8 activation is important to control infected cells. There has been reported a relation between HLA-class I haplotypes and CD8 cellular reponse with prognosis of PML. CD8 cytotoxic lymphocites (CTL) recognise the epitopes of viral proteins presented on the class I HLA molecules of infected cells and eliminate them. Several CTL epitopes have been mapped [7, 8].

Nowadays, the prevalence of PML in the general population was estimated at 4.4 cases per 100000 individuals [7]. PML is most frequent in patients infected with HIV. According to these results, several studies have demonstrated that PML is rare in non-HIV population [11, 12].

PML often progresses during weeks or months, leading to a severe disability and even finally to death [10]. The neurological deficits depend on the localitation of the demyelination areas in the brain. Symptoms can vary and include muscle weakness, hemianopsia, sensory deficits, cognitive dysfunction, aphasia and/or coordination and gait difficulties. The spinal cord and the optic nerves are not usually involved. Patients can present seizures if the lesions are near the cortex [7].

The brain lesions usually are detected by MRI or TC scan, they are frecuently localizated in the white matter and do not correspond to specific vascular areas/territories. The grey matter could be affected too, such as the thalamus or the basal ganglia. TC shows hypodense or patchy areas and in MRI lesions appear as hypointense images on T1-weighted and hyperintense images en T2-weighted and fluid attenuated inversion recovery images. There is not presence of oedema, mass effect or contrast enhacement.

Patients may present multiple lesions and they are usually located in the subcortical hemispheric white matter or the cerebellar peduncles [7]. Contrast enhacement in MRI has been reported to occur in 50% of HIV-infected patients who have relatively long-term survival [4].

The diagnosis is established by detection of JC virus DNA in the cerebrospinal fluid (CSF) by polymerase chain reaction (PCR) or detection of viral DNA or viral proteins by immunohistochemistry or in situ hibridisation on a brain biopsy sample. Several cases with typical clinical and radiological findings might be thought of as possible PML even without JC virus detection in the CSF if other infectious and tumoral causes have been ruled out [7].

The detection of JC virus DNA in CSF by PCR has a sensibility of 72-92% and a specifity of 92-100%. So, it must be considered that a negative result of JC virus PCR does not ruled out PML [8].

Histologically, there are multiple areas of demyelination because of the litic infection of oligodendrocytes and astrocytes. The nuclei of the oligodendrocytes become enlarged and densely basophilic with eosinofilic inclusions. Moreover, bizarre multinucleated astrocytes and reactive gliosis can be observed [7, 8].

PML - Immune Reconstitution Inflamatory Syndrome (IRIS)

A rapid recovery of the immune system is not always favourable and lead to an immune reconstitution inflammatory syndrome (IRIS).

IRIS is observed in HIV-positive patients with PML in treatment with combination antiretroviral therapy [1, 13]. It can be diagnosed when patients present an elevation of CD4 and CD8 T cell counts with decreased HIV RNA levels in plasma and an inflammatory response associated with an acute and transient clinical worsening. Because of that inflammation, enhancing lesions, oedema and sometimes mass effect can be seen in MRI. The detection of JC virus DNA by PCR may be negative related to the recovery of the immune system. It has been described that steroids can benefit in several cases. [1, 7, 9]. Alternatives to corticosteroids have also been proposed, as the use of maraviroc, the CCR5 chemikine receptor antagonist [14].

Risk Factors

It has been described several situations related to development of PML: HIV-infection, hematological malignancies, transplants recipients, autoimmune diseases, chemotherapy and patients in treatment with monoclonal antibodies, which are explained below:

HIV Infection

AIDS is the leading predisposing disease to PML [15]. Since 1980´s when HIV epidemic emerged, PML have become a several complication of HIV infection [10]. In that moment, the incidence increased 50-fold, until the introduction of highly active antiretroviral therapy. Since then, the incidence of PML in HIV patients has decreased and remains between 3-5%. [10]

Highly active antiretroviral therapy (HAART) has improved survival after the diagnosis of PML. Despite of that, prognosis is poor with a high mortality rate and high degree of sequelae among survivors. It has been suggested that cell count of > 200 versus <200 at diagnosis of HIV infection was a marker for a decreased risk to develop PML [2, 5].

So far, a specific treatment is still unknown, so the main objective to management of PML must be avoid immunodeficiency through early diagnosis and treatment of HIV infection.

It has been suggested that those types of HAART with a high CNS penetrance could be effective in treating PML, because these regimens decrease HIV viral load in CNS and could have influence in JC virus replication [5]. A recent publication has described a survival improvement in patients who receive intensive HAART with five drugs, one of them enfuvirtide [16]. Moreover, a multicentre retrospective observational study reports an improvement in survival of a group receiving protease inhibitors with lower mortality rates; so a treatment based on protease inhibitors may be indicated in PML-patients [5].

It has been described a classification developed for Cinque *et al.*, for planning and investigating treatment interventions that uses two components: combined antitretroviral therapy and immunovirological response and inflammatory features [8].

Hematological Malignancies

Since its first description in 1958 by Astrom, in three patients with Hodgkin´s lymphoma and chronic lymphatic leukemia (CLL), most of PML ceases described until early 1980´s were secondary to hematological malignancies. Then, this situation changed in relation to VIH pandemia onset.

Other associated hematological disorders are Non-Hodgkin lymphoma, multiple myeloma, Waldenstrom macroglobulinemia and it has been seen also in patients who have undergone hematopoietic stem cell transplantation (HSCT) [6].

The incidence rate of PML in CLL patients has been 11.1 per 100000 person-years in a recent study published. It was suspected that pathogenetic mechanism was related to a immunodysregulation secondary to the therapy, because most of the patients had a long disease history with multiple treatment regimens. In fact, the relation between purine analogues and monoclonal antibodies with of PML are not umcommon in the literature [6], but there is a controversy because there are few cases of PML in CLL in naïve patients. Therefore more investigations are necessary to elucidate the underlying pathogenical mechanism and to develop efficient treatment strategies [17].

Transplants Recipients

Transplant recipients are at significant risk of developing PML during the immediately posttransplantation period. The first report of PML in a transplant recipient was in 1971. Despite the risk of PML among transplant recipients, clinical characteristics, risk factors and incidence remain yet uncertain. The risk is 1.24 per 1000 posttransplantation person years for heart and lung transplant recipients al one institution with over 98% follow-up. This incidence is comparable with risk in patients with natalizumab, and is higher than HIV-patients treated with HAART and other rheumatologial disorders. The immunosuppressive medication is the principal underlying risk factor in cases of solid organ transplantation. Bone narrow recipients survive longer than solid organ recipients, but have a lower median time to symptom onset because of their level of immunosupression, previous hematologic malignancies and chemotherapy. The case fatality is high and the 1 year-survival is 56% similar to HIV-patients treated with HAART. It is described that among survivors, some patients reduced or withdrawn their immunosuppressive drug regimen at time of PML diagnosis, but no treatment is considered completely effective. The most important determinants for PML development are immunosupression and transplantation and not the underlying disease. To date, the immune reconstitution is the only way to improve transplant recipients diagnosed of PML situation, but a graft rejection may be develop [5].

PML in the setting of hematopoietic cell transplantation is rare [18]. Several cases have been reported in HTC recipients since 1992. It has been described in comparable frequency following both allogeneic and autologous HTC. The incidence among this population is lower than in HIV cases, with incidence rates of 35.4 vs 130 per one hundred thousand person years, respectively. The median time from transplantation to symptom onset has been described as 11 months, shorter than other viral encephalitis in these patients. Published data suggested that the median of survival in those patients that not received any treatment from time of symptoms onset, was two months [19]. HSCT patients with PML presented varying CD4+ counts, from normal to very low at time of diagnosis in contrast with low levels in AIDS patients or those receiving purine analogues. These findings suggest that apart prior treatment-induced immunosupression, other aspects may be considered [6]. On the other hand, a review of different treatment strategies reveals that since 2007 majority of treatment regimens include 5HT2A blockers, which is the site for JC virus binding [19].

Autoimmune Diseases

PML has been described in autoimmune diseases like rheumatoid arthritis (RA), vasculitis, ***systemic*** lupus erythematosus (SLE) or sarcoidosis. It is suggested that spondylarthropathies are not associated with an increased risk of PML [15].

Information from a US database reported a PML prevalence of 0.4/10000 person-year in RA patients which not differ from that in patients without HIV infection. In the largest case-series of PML, 0.25% of patients had RA. In few cases described, patients who presented PML were taking a combination of immunosuppressant medication or a single-drug therapy. On the other hand the prevalence in SLE patients is 4/100000 person-year and based inpublised case-series, 0.44% of patients with PML had SLE. Over 50% were receiving immunosuppressant therapy, mainly azathioprine and cyclophosphamide. However, it is thought that SLE per se may increased the risk of develop PML based on 40 % of patients had received less immunosupressive regimens, the mechanism is unknown, but level of lymphopenia may be involved. In other systemic diseases the prevalence is increased too, especially in vasculitides such Wegener´s granulomatosis and poly-or dermatomiositis. Only a few cases of PML have been recorded in patients with Sjogren´s syndrome or sclerodermia.

There is a low frequency of sarcoidosis associated PML. In 1955, Christensen and Fog described the first association and since then several cases reports have been published. It is suggested that this disorder is not only due to lymphocytopenia or immunosuppressive medications, more complex mechanisms are implicated in. It has been described that patients may be often misdiagnosed, so it leads a management delay. A poor survival rate has been reported compared with other immunosuppressive status associated with PML, because of inappropriate intensification of immunosuppression and difficulty in reverse cell-mediated dysregulation [15].

Natalizumab

Natalizumab is a humanized IgG4 monoclonal antibody against the cell adhesion molecule α4-integrin. Natalizumab is used in the treatment of multiple sclerosis and Chron's disease. Antibodies against α4 integrins inhibit the binding of cells expressing α4β1 integrin and α4β7 integrin (eg, lymphocytes) to vascular-cell adhesion molecule 1 on endothelial cells. This is a crucial step in the movement of T-lymphocytes across the endothelial-cell basal lamina and into the CNS parenchyma [10].

PML has been shown to be highly associated with natalizumab treatment. Actually, natalizumab is the only high PML risk drug that remains on the market. As of 2014, 454 patients diagnosed with confirmed PML (452 with multiple sclerosis and 2 with Crohn disease) had been treated with natalizumab [20].

In 2010, Clifford *et al.* reported 28 cases of confirmed PML in patients with multiple sclerosis treated with natalizumab, of which eight were fatal. The median treatment duration to onset of symptoms was 25 months (range 6-80 months). The presenting symptoms most commonly included changes in cognition, personality, and motor performance, but several cases had seizures as the first clinical event [21].

In a study by Bloomgren *et al.*, they used data from postmarketing sources, clinical studies, and an independent Swedish registry to estimate the incidence of PML among natalizumab-treated patients with multiple sclerosis, according to positive or negative status with respect to anti–JC virus antibodies, prior or no prior use of immunosuppressants, and duration of treatment (1 to 24 months vs. 25 to 48 months). As of February 29, 2012, there were 212 confirmed cases of PML among 99,571 patients treated with natalizumab (2.1 cases per 1000 patients). When the risk of PML was stratified according to three risk factors, the risk of PML was lowest among the patients who were negative for anti–JC virus antibodies, with the incidence estimated to be 0.09 cases or less per 1000 patients (95% confidence interval [CI], 0 to 0.48). Patients who were positive for anti–JC virus antibodies, had taken immunosuppressants before the initiation of natalizumab therapy, and had received 25 to 48 months of natalizumab treatment had the highest estimated risk (incidence, 11.1 cases per 1000 patients [95% CI, 8.3 to 14.5]) [22].

To assess risk factors and quantify the risk of PML in these patients has been necessary. The duration of therapy, prior use of immunosuppressive therapies and anti-JCV antibody status are established risk factors for development of PML in natalizumab-treated patients. The group at lowest risk of developing PML consists of those who tested negative for anti-JCV antibodies, with an estimated PML risk of 0.11 per 1000 patients (95% CI: 0, 0.59). Patients with all three risk factors (i.e. natalizumab treatment for more than 2 years, prior immunosuppressive therapy, and anti-JCV antibody-positive status) had an estimated risk of PML of 7.8 per 1000 patients (95% CI: 5.2, 11.3). However, the most recent risk calculation suggests an increased risk of PML in JCV antibody positive patients Anti-JCV antibody-positive patients with no prior use of immunosuppressants have an estimated risk of developing PML approximately twice as high as the overall natalizumab-treated population, as roughly half of patients with MS are anti-JCV antibody positive [23].

Anti-JCV antibody levels in serum/plasma, measured as index, may differentiate PML risk in anti-JCV antibody-positive multiple sclerosis patients with no prior immunosuppressant use [24]. Other proposed risk factors has recently been JC virus DNA. A spanish study concluded that the determination of JCV DNA levels in urine could be complementary to anti-JCV antibodies for identifying MS patients who has been infected by the JCV [25].

Rituximab

Rituximab is a chimaeric murine/human monoclonal antibody directed against the surface antigen CD20, a lineage specific receptor, being expressed in both, the healthy and the majority of malignant B-cells. Rituximab has been the first monoclonal antibody to be approved by the U.S. Food and Drug Administration to treat cancer. Since its approval, rituximab treatment leads to a significantly increased patients' survival affected by B cell non-Hodgkin lymphoma and has already been widely incorporated into clinical use, as in other areas such as autoimmune diseases [26].

Its infusion results in a rapid depletion of B-cell lymphocytes in peripheral blood, lymph nodes and bone marrow; and the amount of circulating immunoglobulin (Ig) may decrease after the treatment with rituximab.

Rituximab has been associated with viral infectious complications. The pathophysiology after rituximab mAb remains uncertain because its treatment does not result in T-cell depletion, as seen in AIDS. However, it has been suggested that after the B-cell depletion, subsequent repletion of the mature B-lymphocytes population results in expansion of pre-B-lymphocytes harbouring latent JC virus [10].

In 2009, Carson et al. reviewed PML case descriptions among patients treated with rituximab from the Food and Drug Administration, the manufacturer, physicians, and a literature review from 1997 to 2008. Overall, 52 patients with lymphoproliferative disorders, 2 patients with systemic lupus erythematosus, 1 patient with rheumatoid arthritis, 1 patient with an idiopathic autoimmune pancytopenia, and 1 patient with immune thrombocytopenia developed PML after treatment with rituximab and other agents. Other treatments included hematopoietic stem cell transplantation (7 patients), purine analogs (26 patients), or alkylating agents (39 patients). One patient with an autoimmune hemolytic anemia developed PML after treatment with corticosteroids and rituximab, and 1 patient with an autoimmune pancytopenia developed PML after treatment with corticosteroids, azathioprine, and rituximab. Median time from first rituximab dose to PML diagnosis was 16.0 months (range, 1.0-90.0 months) and from last rituximab dose to PML diagnosis was 5.5 months (range, 0.3-66.0 months).

Presenting findings included confusion/disorientation (54% of patients), motor weakness/hemiparesis (33%), poor motor coordination (25%), speech changes (21%), or vision changes (18%). Median duration between last rituximab dose and PML diagnosis was shorter among patients who had CD4+ lymphocyte counts < 500 cells/μL (3 months vs 17 months for patients with CD4+ lymphocyte counts > 500 cells/μL). The case-fatality rate was 90%: 100% among PML cases diagnosed within 3 months of the last rituximab dose versus 84% among PML cases diagnosed more than 3 months after the last rituximab dose. PML treatments included cytarabine or antiviral or immunologic therapies. Of 5 patients who did not die of PML, 2 received no therapy, 1 received cytarabine, another mirtazapine, and the last received cidofovir, donor lymphocyte infusions, cytarabine, and risperidone. These patients had residual neurologic deficits including motor aphasia, hemiparesis, and visual defects [27].

Subsequent studies have estimated the incidence of JC viremia in rituximab-treated solid-organ transplant patients to be at 5.5% [28]. Clifford and co-workers described an increased risk, about 1 case per 25000 individuals with rheumathoid arthritis of PML in patients being treated with rituximab [29].

In an analysis published in 2013 of the incidence of new infections and reactivations of different viruses with individuals receiving rituximab for new onset type 1 diabetes, no JCV reactivations were detected in this study, but among 6 (17%) rituximab and 2 (8%) placebo recipients who seroconverted for JCV during the study, only one rituximab recipient had detectable viremia. All primary infections were asymptomatic [30].

After all this data, a prevalence of rituximab-associated PML is estimated to be < 1/30.000 and because of that, it has been classified as a low PML risk treatment [20].

Efalizumab

Efalizumab is a humanized IgG1 monoclonal antibody that binds CD11a, the α subunit of leucocyte function associated antigen 1 (LFA 1), which bind to intracellular adhesion molecule on antigen-pressenting cells. Blockade of these interactions prevents lymphocyte activation, proliferation and migration. As this process is thought to be an important step in the pathogenesis of skin diseases, efalizumab was investigated in the treatment of moderate to severe psoriasis [10].

Three cases suggest that prolongad efalizumab therapy is a risk factor for PML. Although the cases reported treatment for longer than 3 years, a specific treatment duration that does not place patients at risk for PML has not been defined [31]. Because of these cases, efalizumab was withdrawn from the market in april, 2009.

With natalizumab, efalizumab is the only drug considered of high PML risk by Calabrese *and colleagues* [20].

Most of the efalizumab-treated patients presented with clinical-difficulties and muscle weeknesses, being these symptoms clearly different from PML related to other monoclonal antibodies [7].

Brentuximab

Brentuximab vedotin (BV) is an antibody-drug conjugate composed of a CD30-directed monoclonal antibody that is covalently linked to the antimicrotubule agent monomethyl auristatin E (MMAE). It has been recently approved by Federal Drug Authority (FDA) and European Medicines Agency (EMA) for treatment of recurrent or refractory anaplastic large cell lymphoma and classic Hodgkin's disease.

PML has been reported in patients who received this treatment alter receiving multiple prior chemotherapy regimens. Prior immunosuppressive therapy and compromised immune systems were postulated risk factors [32].

Recently, a work by Carson *et al.* have described a report of 5 HIV-negative cases who developed BV-associated PML. Indications for BV were classic Hodgking lymphoma in 3 patients, and 2 immunocompetent patients diagnosed of cutaneous T-cell lymphomas without prior chemotherapy:1 with a primary cutaneous anaplastic large cell lymphoma and 1 with a transformed mycosis fungoides [33].

Time to the onset of symptoms and duration of therapy before PML has been described to be shorter in patients treated with BV than in patients treated with other monoclonal antibodies, as rituximab, natalizumab or efalizumab. PML developed after a median of 3 doses (range, 2 doses-6 doses) and within a media of 7 weeks after BV iniatiation (range, 3 weeks-34 weeks). Four patients died at a median of 8 weeks after the diagnosis. The sole survivor was started on prednisone after interruption BV. She represents the first case of PML-IRIS after BV or rituximab with a previous diagnosis of a lymphoma, and demostrated slow but definite improvement [34].

Further investigations on mechanisms of PML causation by brentuximab are warranted, being suggested that depletion of CD30-expressing activated T cells could reduce JCV immune surveillance in the central nervous system, resulting in PML.

Alemtuzumab

Alemtuzumab is a monoclonal antibod that binds to CD52, an antigen expressed on the surface of mature B and T lymphocytes, but not on the stem cells. After treatment with alemtuzumab, these lymphocytes are targeted for lysis.

This drug is used in the treatment of chronic lymphocytic leukemia (CLL), cutaneous T-cell lymphoma, peripheral T-cell lymphomas (PTCL) and in the treatment of multiple sclerosis. It has been used in organ and stem cell transplantation.

Only three cases of PML have been reported to date: one patient after 3 months of treatment for CLL, another with a PTCL who received alemtuzumab after 8 cycles of CHOP, and a third in a lung transplant recipiente who received steroids, anti-thymocyte glubulin and alemtuzumab [35].

TNF Inhibitors: Infliximab, Etanercept and Adalimumab

Anti-tumor necrosis factor (TNF)-alpha drugs are a class of drugs that have ben used for more than 10 years. They are used worldwide to their inflammatory conditions such as rheumatoid arthritis, psoriatic arthritis, juvenile arthritis, Chron´s disease, ulcerative colitis, ankylosing spondylitis and psoriasis.

There are five anti-TNF drugs that have been approved by the U.S. Food and Drug Administration: infliximab, etanercept, adalimumab, certolizumab and golimumab.

Despite this spread use, recent publications [20, 36] have classified them in the group of very low risk of drugs with which this disease has been related because the few cases reported. Actually, PML risk is confounded by the use of other immunosupresive agents.

JC virus reactivation risk has been investigated in patients after been treated with infliximab. Peripheral mononuclear blood cells (PBMC), plasma and urine samples were obtained from 61 immune-mediated diseases patients treated or not with infliximab in combination with steroid and other immunomodulators and from 20 healthy donors. JCV DNA was transiently detected in 12 PBMC of 40 patients at different doses of infliximab with a higher prevalence than that of the 21 patients untreated. Conversely, a stable JCV positivity in urine of treated and untreated patients was detected. Sequencing the noncoding control region (NCCR), all samples exhibited the archetype structure with few mutations in transcriptional factor binding regions. The consequence of anti-TNF-α treatment on viral persistence was examined monitoring Torquetenovirus viremia and investigating the TNF-α-induced microRNA regulators of transcriptional factors, with a binding site on NCCR. Infliximab treatment in this study did not affect directly JCV reactivation [37].

Just a few cases have been comunicated. In a finnish work with 23 children with severe inflammatory bowel disease, 141 infliximab infusions were patterned in the follow-up period. A severe adverse reaction in a 16-year old boy after the second infliximab infusion, with radiologycal changes similar to PML, with no specific findings in biopsy and without an infective agent found was reported [38].

Other cases as the one with an adult man with rheumathoid arthritis whose symptoms developed after 3 years of treatment have been published [39].

Case reports related to etanercept and adalimumab have also been comunicated is patients with different autoimmune diseases [40-42].

Fingolimod

Fingolimod is an immunomodulating drug for the treatment of multiple sclerosis. It is the first oral disease-modifying drug for the treatment of relapsing forms of multiple sclerosis.

This mechanism of action of fingolimod is base don an antagonic effect on the sphingosine-1-phosphate receptors that will generate an inhibition of the egress of naive and central memory lymphoytes into the bloodstream, allowing the free recirculation of memory effectors T lymphocytes. This effect will thus produce lymphopenia. Fingolimod-associated lymphopenia is a consequence of lymphocyte redistribution [43].

Almost all leukoencephalopathy cases on fingolimod have received previous natalizumab. Several cases of patients requiering treatment for multiple sclerosis with natalizumab-associated PML have been reported [44].

A recent study evaluating the efficacy of fingolimod to treat severe multiple sclerosis after natalizumab-associated PML suggests that using fingolimod for these high-risk patients may be an option, under close clinical and radiological monitoring [45].

It has also been suggested a theoretical risk of PML if natalizumab is transiently combined with another immune-altering agent and the value of transiently "reconstituting" CNS immune surveillance by washout of natalizumab in an effort to clear theoretical subclinical JC virus within the CNS. The optimal length of natalizumab washout became the subject of intense consternation and debate, with no clear guidelines to inform practice. However, upon withdrawing natalizumab, resumption of disease activity was soon observed, beginning 3-4 months after the last dose of natalizumab. Postnatalizumab return of disease raised concern that the washout may harm the patient by a severe relapse with incomplete recovery [46].

Ruxolitinib

Ruxolitinib is a JAK 1 and JAK 2 inhibitor approved for the treatment of disease-related splenomegaly or symptoms in adult patients with primary myelofybrosis (also known as chronic idiopathic myelofybrosis), post-polycythemia vera myelofibrosis or post-essential thrombocythemia myelofibrosis.

As JAK-STAT pathway has an important role in host defense and autoimmunity, JAK inhibition can lead to lethal viral and bacterial infection.

A 75-year-old man with intermediate-2-risk myelofibrosis that was refractory to hidroxiurea therapy has been communicated to receive ruxolitinib. Ten weeks after therapy was initiated, he started with cognitive impairment and worsening expressive dysphasia. Over the following weeks, the symptoms progressed with a brain biopsy after several tests consistent with PML [47].

Belimumab

Belimumab is a human monoclonal antibody that inhibits B-cell activating factor, or BAFF, also known as B-lymphocyte stimulator (BLyS). Belimumab was approved by the FDA in 2011 for patients with systemic lupus erythematosus who failed after standard therapy.

A case of PML in a lupus 40 year-old woman has been also reported after a total of 10 infusions of belimumab [48].

Table 1. Immunomodulatory agents associated with PML

Immunomodulatory agent	Mechanism of action
Natalizumab	Anti - α4-integrin mAb
Rituximab	Anti - CD20 mAb
Efalizumab	Anti - CD11 mAb
Brentuximab	Anti - CD30 mAb
Alemtuzumab	Anti-CD52
Infliximab	Anti - TNFα
Etanercept	Anti - TNFα
Adalimumab	Anti - TNFα
Fingolimod	Sphingosine-1-phosphate receptor modulator
Ruxolitinib	JAK 1 and 2 inhibitor
Belimumab	Anti - BAFF

Management Strategies

There is no proven treatment with proven efficiency. Development of an effective antiviral therapy has been challenging due to the absence of an animal model of PML because the JC virus is a neurotropic virus that infects only human beings. Aditionally, there have been also difficulties trying to propagate JC virus in human cell cultures, despite binding to the serotoninergic 5-HT2a receptor to infect astroglial cells in vitro [7, 14].

While different antiviral or immunomodulant medications have been proposed or even used for the treatment of PML, none has proven real effective. Most of these drugs have been evaluated in retrospective series or groups of case reports.

The treatment strategies include antineoplastic agents, as cytarabine and topotecan; antiviral drugs, as cidofovir; immunomodulant agents, as □-interferon, □-interferon or interleukin-2; and antidepressants, as serotonin antagonists like mirtazapine. The last drug investigated was mefloquine, that has been extensively used for prophylaxis and treatment of malaria.

Cytarabine arabinoside, also known as ara-C, is an anti-metabolite normally used to treat acute leucemias and non-Hodgkin lymphomas, and instead of cytidine, is incorporated into DNA, leading to competitive inhibition of the DNA polymerase and thus to the inhibition of DNA synthesis. It has been shown to inhibit JC virus replication and multiplication *in vitro* in a persistently infected human fetal brain cell line [49].

Some isolated reports and the *in vitro* activity support its investigation as a drug with activity against JC virus [50, 51]. A spanish report with 13 HIV patients with biopsy proven PML revealed only modest short-term clinical improvement in the conditions of patients treated with the drug, with no significant impact on survival, with a median survival time after diagnosis of 102 days (range, 46-220 days) for 8 patients who received cytarabine and 60 days (range, 28-72) for 5 untreated patients [52].

A multicenter trial testing ara-C in 57 patients with HIV-associated and biopsy-proven PML were randomly assigned to receive antiretroviral therapy alone, antiretroviral therapy plus intravenous cytarabine, or antiretroviral therapy plus intrathecal cytarabine, with median survival times of 11, 8 and 5 weeks, respectively. Because of these results, it was concluded that cytarabine administered either intravenously or intrathecally does not improve the prognosis of HIV-infected patients with PML [53].

Cytosine arabinoside given intravenously to non-AIDS PML patients in an open label small study with 19 patients was associated with a 36% chance of developing stabilization at 1 year [54].

Topotecan, a topoisomerase I inhibitor, is a water-soluble derivative of camptothecin. JC virus DNA replication requires the viral early protein T-antigen and host-replication factors including DNA polymerases and DNA topoisomerase I. In an in vitro study, Kerr et al. were able to block replication of viral DNA in glial cells using camptothecin, demonstrating that repeated pulse-treatment of cells with the drug is required for complete blockage of viral DNA replication [55].

In a phase II clinical trial with topotecan administered to a cohort of 11 subjects with AIDS-related PML, three patients were treatment responders, showing a neurological improvement. Despite the results, the study was too small to provide conclusive information about the drug's efficacy [56].

Cidofovir is an antiviral drug used to treat cytomegalovirus retinitis in AIDS-people. It has been shown to inhibit replication of mouse polyomavirus and SV40 in vitro [8]. Initially, most case reports shown that the drug was effective. Cidofovir was suggested to be the most reasonable treatment option for PML in HIV-patients who fail to improve with HAART or who were unable to tolerate these regimens [57].

The analysis of raw data from one prospective and five cohort studies by De Luca et al. concluded that in combination with antiretroviral therapy, cidofovir use did not influence PML-related mortality (Hazard ratio for death 0.93; 95% CI 0.66-1.32) or residual disability by 12 months [58].

One case report of an apparently immunocompetent patient with PML had an obvious benefit of treatment with cidofovir [59].

Biological activity has been suggested for interpheron alpha and beta (alpha-IFN and beta-IFN) in PML. Interferons belong to the large class of proteins known as cytokines, with antiviral and immunomodulant activities.

A retrospective chart review was conducted to determine the effect of alpha-IFN in 77 patients with HIV-associated PML at the John Hopkins Hospital between 1985 and 1986. Among deceased patients, median survival of treated patients was 127.5 days longer than that of untreated patients (Chi-square=4.21, p=0.04) and when living and deceased patientes were combined, the median survival was 325 days (range 35-1634 days) versus 121 days (range 46-176) in untreated patients (Chi-square=13.47, p<0.001). In addition, use of alpha-IFN was associated with a significant delay in the Honest of memory loss (Chi-square=8.59, p<0.001). In conclusion, this study suggests that alpha-IFN may delay progression, palliate symptoms, and significantly prolong survival in this subgroup of patients [60].

A subsequent retrospective study exploring the roles of HAART and alpha-IFN in improving survival of patients with AIDS-related PML analyzed 97 patients. Multivariate analysis showed greater survival for those on HAART. Whereas IFN-alpha use was shown to be associated with longer survival (p<0.057), this effect was not independent of the effects of HAART. Consequently, IFN-alpha did not appeared ti provide adicional benefit [61].

IFN-beta has also a number of antiviral effects. A case report of a patient with HIV infection and PML has been published after being treated with IFN-beta, but the neurologic course progressed despite treatment [62].

Other cytokines have been focused in the therapeutics of PML like interleukin 2 (IL-2), an immunomodulant protein that is important for the proliferation of T and B lymphocytes and other activities crucial to regulation of the immune response.

Because a plausible biological basis exists for a role for recombinant IL-2 in the reconstitution of impaired antiviral immune functions, diverse data with patients has been published. A patient with low-grade lymphoma treated with IL-2 resulted in near complete resolution of symptoms and MRI abnormalities, with an absolute Lumber of CD3+ CD4+ also increased and the CD4/CD8 ratio normalized, remaining free of evidence of PML 1 year off therapy [63].

However, a later report of a patient with myelodysplasia who developed PML showed an improvement in his neurological functions, despite remaining severely lymphopenic with a low absolute CD3 CD4+ cell count despite a clinical response to treatment [64].

Recently, it has been found that the serotoninergic receptor 5HT2a receptor could act as the cellular receptor for JC virus on human glial cells. This highlights the possibility that serotonine receptor antagonists, as mirtazapine, may be useful in the treatment of PML [65].

Although a possible benefit has been proposed in most of reported cases with patients inffected with HIV [66] or with haematologycal malignancies [67], there is no sufficient evidence to recommend treatment as a standard.

A study published by Marzocchetti et al. reported that 14 patients with PML (7 HIV+ and 7 HIV -) treated with mirtazapine within 1 year after PML diagnosis was compared with 11 patients with PML (6 HIV+ and 5 HIV -) who were not receiving any other treatment except HAART. The 1-year survival rate was 62% in patients treated with the serotonina receptor blocker versus 45% in untreated patients (HR for death 0.63, 95% CI 0.19-2.07, p=0.45) [68].

There is also one case report of a 33-year-old comatose haploidentical stem cell transplant recipient treated with risperidone, another serotonine 2A receptor, achieveing a clinical, neuroradiological and virological response [69].

The most recent therapy tested was the antimalarial mefloquine. This agent was selected between 2000 approved drugs and biologically active molecules for their anti-JC virus activities in an in vitro infection assay. Of the compounds with anti-JC virus activities, only mefloquine has been reported to show sufficiently high penetration into the central servous system [70]. It was demonstrated that mefloquine does not to block viral cell entry; rather, it inhibits viral replication in cells after viral entry.

As mefloquine is a extesively used drug, due to its safety and the urgent need for better therapy for PML, some studies have been organizad to test its activity. Clifford et al. found that mefloquine did not show evidence of in vivo antiviral activity against JC virus as evaluated by JCV DNA load in cerebrospinal fluid (CSF) or clinical / MRI findings. A decrease in CSF JCV DNA load from baseline to week 4 was associated with a better clinical outcome at 16 weeks [71].

Combination of drugs have also been proposed in several case reports. Dual therapy with cidofovir and mirtazapine for progressive PML in a sarcoidosis patient has shown significant improvement of neurological symptoms without measurable functional deficit [72].

Two patients who developed PML, one after HIV and one after allogeneic hematopoietic cell transplantation were treated with the combination of mefloquine and mirtazapine, showing a favorable improvement in clinical symptoms and imaging findings [73, 74], while a favorable outcome were reported in two patients with dermatomyositis treated with cytarabine and mirtazapine [75].

With regard to prophylaxis, neither pre-exposure prophylaxis nor post-exposure is possible [76]. However, mirtazapine has been proposed also as a prophylaxis agent [66].

Without a specific antiviral drug, the mainstay of therapy remains to be the immune reconstitution. In HIV patients, this immune reconstitution should be based on HAART. However, between HIV-negative patients, the objective should be based, when possible, on reducing the immunosupressant drugs. Given the expanding population at risk and the high mortality of PML, an effective therapy has become an important research goal.

PROGNOSIS

From 1958 to 1980´s PML was observed in patients treated with immunosuppressive medication, mainly in hematological malignancies. When AIDS emerged, the incidence increased 50-fold and HIV infection becomes the main predisposing condition to develop PML. In the pre-highly active antiretroviral therapy (HAART) era, up to 5% of HIV patients presented PML, the median survival was 6 months and 1 year-survival since the onset of the symptoms was less than 10% [12].

Almost 4700 patients from a nationwide population-based cohort of adult HIV-1-infected individuals were included in a nationwide cohort study during the period before highly active antiretroviral therapy (HAART) (1995-1996) and during the early HAART (1997-1999) and late HAART (2000-2006).

They reported incidence rates to be 3.3, 1.8, and 1.3 cases per 1000 person-years at risk in 1995-1996, 1997-1999, and 2000-2006, respectively, and median survival times were 0.4 years (95% confidence interval [CI], 0.0-0.7) in 1995-1996 and 1.8 years (95% CI, 0.6-3.0) in both 1997-1999 and 2000-2006 [2].

Data from a Swiss cohort showed a decrease of the incidence from 0.24 cases per 1000 patient-year before HAART era to 0.06 cases per 100 patient-years after introduction of HAART. In a Danish cohort, the incidence rate was 1.3 cases per 1000 person-years [11] and the EuroSIDA cohort showed an important decrease in the incidence from 10 to 1 case per 1000 person-year between 1995 and 2001 [77]. PML mortality has decreased since the mid-1990´s when HAART became the standard therapy, resulting in an improvement of the survival among this group of patients [77].

PML is typically associated with minimal inflammation; however, patients may develop an inflammatory response due to IRIS. A retrospective review by Harrison et al. was performed on 87 patients diagnosed with PML at Johns Hopkins, 27 of which had a syndrome consistent with IRIS. Gadolinium enhancement on MRI occurred in 44.4% of cases of PML-IRIS versus 5.1% in PML ($p<0.05$), and thus had low diagnostic sensitivity and specificity. In HIV+ cases, CD4 counts were lower in those who later developed IRIS (mean 34.8 vs. 71.7, $p<0.05$) and was predictive of the development of IRIS ($p<0.05$). Improved prognosis was seen with higher CSF white blood cell counts and protein levels, but not for gadolinium enhancement and there were no differences in survival for PML versus PML-IRIS [78].

Other multicenter, open-label pilot trial evaluated the survival benefit of a five-drug combined HAART designed to accelerate HIV replication decay and JC virus specific immune recovery, as 50% of patients have told to be died within 6 months after the symptoms begin. 28 patients received an optimized cART with three or more drugs for 12 months, plus the fusion inhibitor enfuvirtide during the first 6 months.

At entry, median CD4+ T-cell count was 53 per microliter and 86% of patients had detectable plasma HIV RNA and CSF JCV DNA levels. Seven patients died, all before month 4. The one-year survival estimate was 0.75 (95% confidence interval, 0.61 to 0.93). At month 6, JCV DNA was undetectable in the CSF of 81% of survivors. At month 12, 81% of patients had undetectable plasma HIV RNA, and the median CD4+ T-cell increment was 105 per microliter. In univariate analysis, higher total and naive CD4+ T-cell counts and lower CSF JCV DNA level at baseline were associated with better survival. JCV-specific functional memory CD4+ T-cell responses, based on a proliferation assay, were detected in 4% of patients at baseline and 43% at month 12 (P=0.008). Therefore, the authors concluded that the early use of five-drug cART after PML diagnosis appears to improve survival, being associated with recovery of anti-JCV T-cell responses and JCV clearance from CSF. A low CD4+ T-cell count (particularly naive subset) and high JCV DNA copies in CSF at PML diagnosis was suggested to be risk factors for death [16].

Between HIV-negative patients affected by lymphoproliferative disorders (LPD) who developed progressive multifocal leukoencephalopathy (PML), García- Suarez and coworkers analyzed whether the new antineoplastic therapies are changing the natural history of this infectious disease.

They communicate a retrospectively analysis of 46 cases with confirmed LPD-associated PML published from 1958 to 2004. Patients were stratified according to two different time periods: group A included patients diagnosed before 1989, and group B included patients diagnosed since 1990, after introduction of purine analogues. Group A patients (n = 22) had received alkylating agents and/or radiotherapy, and the majority (63.6%) had advanced Hodgkin disease. At univariate analysis, uncontrolled Hodgkin disease was the only risk factor for PML. In group B patients (n = 24), the most frequent treatments received were purine analogues (58.3%) and high-dose therapy with hematopoietic stem cell transplantation (33.3%; HDT/HSCT). B-CLL (45.8%) and aggressive non-Hodgkin lymphoma (24.9%) were the most frequent underlying LPDs. Patients treated with purine analogues were more likely to have active LPD, lower CD4 cell counts, and to be older and male than were HSCT recipients. The median interval from purine analogues or HDT/HSCT to PML was 11 months. In HDT/HSCT recipients, this interval was delayed for 10 months when peri-transplantation rituximab was used. Univariate analysis identified age >55 years, male sex, and CD4 cell counts <or=0.2 x 10(9)/L as risk factors for PML in patients treated with purine analogues. Mortality rates were 95.4% (group A patients), 90% (purine analogues), and 62.5% (HDT/HSCT recipients). At univariate analysis, the only factor that significantly correlated with recovery from infection was female sex. Their findings indicate the possible reduction in reported cases associated with Hodgkin disease and the increasing number of published cases associated with the new antineoplastic therapies (purine analogues and HDT/HSCT); among patients treated with purine analogues, PML is more common in male patients with CD4 cell counts <or=0.2 x 10(9)/L; the use of rituximab after HDT/HSCT seems to delay the onset of PML; and the prognosis is slightly better in transplant recipients [79].

However, and contrary to the previously reported, Clifford [14] confirmed that transplant patients and postchemotherapy patients have a much worse prognosis, as well as being a complex clinical study population due to multiple simultaneous medical complications.

Conclusion

Progressive multifocal leukoencephalopathy is a serious and usually fatal demyelinating disease of the CNS caused by the John Cunningham virus, that can occur in severely immunosupressed patients.

CD4 and CD8 T cells lymphopenia, HIV infection, chemotherapy or immunosupressive therapies related to solid organ transplants, and the most important risk factors. Since their introduction, monoclonal antibodies and immunomodulant agents have found an expanding role in the treatment of cancer and several autoimmune diseases, mainly. Despite their global use, some of them, specially natalizumab, efalizumab and rituximab, have been closely related to PML being a main reason for pharmacovigilance throughout the life cycle of these products.

As any antiviral drug for JC virus causing PML has been deveoped, several therapies have been used for these patients trying to improve their bad life expectancy. Despite all the efforts, immune reconstitution is still considered to be the most practical approach.

Rferences

[1] Weissert R. Progressive multifocal leukoencephalopathy. *J Neuroimmunol.* 2011 Feb;231(1-2):73–7.

[2] Engsig FN, Hansen A-BE, Omland LH, Kronborg G, Gerstoft J, Laursen AL, et al. Incidence, clinical presentation, and outcome of progressive multifocal leukoencephalopathy in HIV-infected patients during the highly active antiretroviral therapy era: a nationwide cohort study. *J Infect Dis.* 2009 Jan 1;199(1):77–83.

[3] Palazzo E, Yahia SA. Progressive multifocal leukoencephalopathy in autoimmune diseases. *Joint Bone Spine.* 2012 Jul;79(4):351–5.

[4] Dworkin MS. A review of progressive multifocal leukoencephalopathy in persons with and without AIDS. *Curr Clin Top Infect Dis.* 2002;22:181–95.

[5] Fanjul F, Riveiro-Barciela M, Gonzalez J, Delgado E, Murillas J, Payeras Cifré A, et al. Evaluation of progressive multifocal leukoencephalopathy treatments in a Spanish cohort of HIV-infected patients: do protease inhibitors improve survival regardless of central nervous system penetration-effectiveness (CPE) score? *HIV Med.* 2013 May;14(5):321–5.

[6] D'Souza A, Wilson J, Mukherjee S, Jaiyesimi I. Progressive multifocal leukoencephalopathy in chronic lymphocytic leukemia: a report of three cases and review of the literature. *Clin Lymphoma Myeloma Leuk.* 2010 Feb;10(1):E1–9.

[7] Tan CS, Koralnik IJ. Progressive multifocal leukoencephalopathy and other disorders caused by JC virus: clinical features and pathogenesis. *Lancet Neurol.* 2010 Apr;9(4):425–37.

[8] Cinque P, Koralnik IJ, Gerevini S, Miro JM, Price RW. Progressive multifocal leukoencephalopathy in HIV-1 infection. *Lancet Infect Dis.* 2009 Oct;9(10):625–36.

[9] Mateen FJ, Muralidharan R, Carone M, van de Beek D, Harrison DM, Aksamit AJ, et al. Progressive multifocal leukoencephalopathy in transplant recipients. *Ann Neurol.* 2011 Aug;70(2):305–22.

[10] Carson KR, Focosi D, Major EO, Petrini M, Richey EA, West DP, et al. Monoclonal antibody-associated progressive multifocal leucoencephalopathy in patients treated with rituximab, natalizumab, and efalizumab: a Review from the Research on Adverse Drug Events and Reports (RADAR) Project. *Lancet Oncol.* 2009 Aug;10(8):816–24.

[11] Amend KL, Turnbull B, Foskett N, Napalkov P, Kurth T, Seeger J. Incidence of progressive multifocal leukoencephalopathy in patients without HIV. *Neurology.* 2010 Oct 12;75(15):1326–32.

[12] Lima MA. Progressive multifocal leukoencephalopathy: new concepts. *Arq Neuropsiquiatr.* 2013 Sep;71(9B):699–702.

[13] Corti M, Villafañe M, Trione N, Yampolsky C, Sevlever G. Progressive multifocal leukoencephalopathy presenting as IRIS in an AIDS patient. A case report and literature review. *Neuroradiol J.* 2013 Apr;26(2):151–4.

[14] Clifford DB. Progressive multifocal leukoencephalopathy therapy. *J Neurovirol.* 2014 Sep 17;

[15] Jamilloux Y, Néel A, Lecouffe-Desprets M, Fèvre A, Kerever S, Guillon B, et al. Progressive multifocal leukoencephalopathy in patients with sarcoidosis. *Neurology.* 2014 Apr 15;82(15):1307–13.
[16] Gasnault J, Costagliola D, Hendel-Chavez H, Dulioust A, Pakianather S, Mazet A-A, et al. Improved survival of HIV-1-infected patients with progressive multifocal leukoencephalopathy receiving early 5-drug combination antiretroviral therapy. *PLoS ONE.* 2011;6(6):e20967.
[17] Di Pauli F, Berger T, Walder A, Maier H, Rhomberg P, Uprimny C, et al. Progressive multifocal leukoencephalopathy complicating untreated chronic lymphatic leukemia: case report and review of the literature. *J Clin Virol.* 2014 Aug;60(4):424–7.
[18] Kharfan-Dabaja MA, Ayala E, Greene J, Rojiani A, Murtagh FR, Anasetti C. Two cases of progressive multifocal leukoencephalopathy after allogeneic hematopoietic cell transplantation and a review of the literature. *Bone Marrow Transplant.* 2007 Jan;39(2):101–7.
[19] Kaufman GP, Aksamit AJ, Klein CJ, Yi ES, Delone DR, Litzow MR. Progressive multifocal leukoencephalopathy: a rare infectious complication following allogeneic hematopoietic cell transplantation (HCT*). Eur J Haematol.* 2014 Jan;92(1):83–7.
[20] Calabrese LH, Molloy E, Berger J. Sorting out the risks in progressive multifocal leukoencephalopathy. *Nat Rev Rheumatol.* 2014 Oct 14;
[21] Clifford DB, De Luca A, DeLuca A, Simpson DM, Arendt G, Giovannoni G, et al. Natalizumab-associated progressive multifocal leukoencephalopathy in patients with multiple sclerosis: lessons from 28 cases. *Lancet Neurol*. 2010 Apr;9(4):438–46.
[22] Bloomgren G, Richman S, Hotermans C, Subramanyam M, Goelz S, Natarajan A, et al. Risk of natalizumab-associated progressive multifocal leukoencephalopathy. *N Engl J Med.* 2012 May 17;366(20):1870–80.
[23] Sørensen PS, Bertolotto A, Edan G, Giovannoni G, Gold R, Havrdova E, et al. Risk stratification for progressive multifocal leukoencephalopathy in patients treated with natalizumab. *Mult Scler.* 2012 Feb;18(2):143–52.
[24] Plavina T, Subramanyam M, Bloomgren G, Richman S, Pace A, Lee S, et al. Anti-JC virus antibody levels in serum or plasma further define risk of natalizumab-associated progressive multifocal leukoencephalopathy. *Ann Neurol.* 2014 Dec;76(6):802–12.
[25] Dominguez-Mozo MI, Garcia-Montojo M, De Las Heras V, Garcia-Martinez A, Arias-Leal AM, Casanova I, et al. Anti-JCV antibodies detection and JCV DNA levels in PBMC, serum and urine in a cohort of

Spanish Multiple Sclerosis patients treated with natalizumab. *J Neuroimmune Pharmacol.* 2013 Dec;8(5):1277–86.

[26] Méndez M and Provencio M. 2013. Rituximab: Pharmacology, clinical indications and health benefits. In: Lake-Bakaar GV, ed. *Rituximab: Pharmacology, clinical indications and health effects.* New York, NY, USA. Nova Science Publishers, pp. 1-30

[27] Kroll JL, Beam C, Li S, Viscidi R, Dighero B, Cho A, et al. Reactivation of latent viruses in individuals receiving rituximab for new onset type 1 diabetes. *J Clin Virol.* 2013 Jun;57(2):115–9.

[28] Clifford DB, Ances B, Costello C, Rosen-Schmidt S, Andersson M, Parks D, et al. Rituximab-associated progressive multifocal leukoencephalopathy in rheumatoid arthritis. *Arch Neurol.* 2011 Sep;68(9):1156–64.

[29] Kamar N, Mengelle C, Rostaing L. Incidence of JC-virus replication after rituximab therapy in solid-organ transplant patients. *Am J Transplant.* 2009 Jan;9(1):244–5.

[30] Carson KR, Evens AM, Richey EA, Habermann TM, Focosi D, Seymour JF, et al. Progressive multifocal leukoencephalopathy after rituximab therapy in HIV-negative patients: a report of 57 cases from the Research on Adverse Drug Events and Reports project. *Blood.* 2009 May 14;113(20):4834–40.

[31] Kothary N, Diak I-L, Brinker A, Bezabeh S, Avigan M, Dal Pan G. Progressive multifocal leukoencephalopathy associated with efalizumab use in psoriasis patients. *J Am Acad Dermatol.* 2011 Sep;65(3):546–51.

[32] Jalan P, Mahajan A, Pandav V, Bekker S, Koirala J. Brentuximab associated progressive multifocal leukoencephalopathy. *Clin Neurol Neurosurg.* 2012 Dec;114(10):1335–7.

[33] Carson KR, Newsome SD, Kim EJ, Wagner-Johnston ND, von Geldern G, Moskowitz CH, et al. Progressive multifocal leukoencephalopathy associated with brentuximab vedotin therapy: a report of 5 cases from the Southern Network on Adverse Reactions (SONAR) project. *Cancer.* 2014 Aug 15;120(16):2464–71.

[34] Von Geldern G, Pardo CA, Calabresi PA, Newsome SD. PML-IRIS in a patient treated with brentuximab. *Neurology.* 2012 Nov 13;79(20): 2075–7.

[35] Berger JR, Houff SA, Major EO. Monoclonal antibodies and progressive multifocal leukoencephalopathy. *MAbs.* 2009 Dec;1(6):583–9.

[36] Chahin S, Berger JR. A risk classification for immunosuppressive treatment-associated progressive multifocal leukoencephalopathy. *J Neurovirol.* 2014 Nov 18;

[37] Giannecchini S, Clausi V, Vultaggio A, Macera L, Maggi F, Martelli F, et al. Assessment of the risk of polyomavirus JC reactivation in patients with immune-mediated diseases during long-term treatment with infliximab. *J Neurovirol.* 2012 Feb;18(1):55–61.

[38] Kolho K-L, Ruuska T, Savilahti E. Severe adverse reactions to Infliximab therapy are common in young children with inflammatory bowel disease. *Acta Paediatr.* 2007 Jan;96(1):128–30.

[39] Kumar D, Bouldin TW, Berger RG. A case of progressive multifocal leukoencephalopathy in a patient treated with infliximab. *Arthritis Rheum.* 2010 Nov;62(11):3191–5.

[40] Graff-Radford J, Robinson MT, Warsame RM, Matteson EL, Eggers SDZ, Keegan BM. Progressive multifocal leukoencephalopathy in a patient treated with etanercept. *Neurologist.* 2012 Mar;18(2):85–7.

[41] Yamamoto M, Takahashi H, Wakasugi H, Sukawa Y, Saito M, Suzuki C, et al. Leukoencephalopathy during administration of etanercept for refractory rheumatoid arthritis. *Mod Rheumatol.* 2007;17(1):72–4.

[42] Ray M, Curtis JR, Baddley JW. A case report of progressive multifocal leucoencephalopathy (PML) associated with adalimumab. *Ann Rheum Dis.* 2014 Jul;73(7):1429–30.

[43] Cervera C. [Infections and fingolimod]. *Rev Neurol.* 2012 Aug 16;55(4):227–37.

[44] Peaureaux D, Pignolet B, Biotti D, Bucciarelli F, Gaina J, Bucur C, et al. Fingolimod treatment after natalizumab-related progressive multifocal leukoencephalopathy: Three new cases. *Mult Scler.* 2014 Oct 10;

[45] Maillart E, Louapre C, Lubetzki C, Papeix C. Fingolimod to treat severe multiple sclerosis after natalizumab-associated progressive multifocal leukoencephalopathy: a valid option? *Mult Scler.* 2014 Apr;20(4):505–9.

[46] Giovannoni G, Naismith RT. Natalizumab to fingolimod washout in patients at risk of PML: when good intentions yield bad outcomes. *Neurology.* 2014 Apr 8;82(14):1196–7.

[47] Wathes R, Moule S, Milojkovic D. Progressive multifocal leukoencephalopathy associated with ruxolitinib. *N Engl J Med.* 2013 Jul 11;369(2):197–8.

[48] Fredericks C, Kvam K, Bear J, Crabtree G, Josephson S. A case of progressive multifocal leukoencephalopathy in a lupus patient treated with belimumab. *Lupus.* 2014 Feb 14;

[49] Hou J, Major EO. The efficacy of nucleoside analogs against JC virus multiplication in a persistently infected human fetal brain cell line. *J Neurovirol.* 1998 Aug;4(4):451–6.

[50] Nicoli F, Chave B, Peragut JC, Gastaut JL. Efficacy of cytarabine in progressive multifocal leucoencephalopathy in AIDS. *Lancet.* 1992 Feb 1;339(8788):306.

[51] Portegies P, Algra PR, Hollak CE, Prins JM, Reiss P, Valk J, et al. Response to cytarabine in progressive multifocal leucoencephalopathy in AIDS. *Lancet.* 1991 Mar 16;337(8742):680–1.

[52] Moreno S, Miralles P, Díaz MD, Berenguer J, Bernaldo de Quirós JC, Blázquez R, et al. Cytarabine therapy for progressive multifocal leukoencephalopathy in patients with AIDS. *Clin Infect Dis.* 1996 Nov;23(5):1066–8.

[53] Hall CD, Dafni U, Simpson D, Clifford D, Wetherill PE, Cohen B, et al. Failure of Cytarabine in Progressive Multifocal Leukoencephalopathy Associated with Human Immunodeficiency Virus Infection. *New England Journal of Medicine.* 1998 May 7;338(19):1345–51.

[54] Aksamit AJ. Treatment of non-AIDS progressive multifocal leukoencephalopathy with cytosine arabinoside. *J Neurovirol.* 2001 Aug;7(4):386–90.

[55] Kerr DA, Chang CF, Gordon J, Bjornsti MA, Khalili K. Inhibition of human neurotropic virus (JCV) DNA replication in glial cells by camptothecin. *Virology.* 1993 Oct;196(2):612–8.

[56] Royal W, Dupont B, McGuire D, Chang L, Goodkin K, Ernst T, et al. Topotecan in the treatment of acquired immunodeficiency syndrome-related progressive multifocal leukoencephalopathy. *J Neurovirol.* 2003 Jun;9(3):411–9.

[57] Segarra-Newnham M, Vodolo KM. Use of cidofovir in progressive multifocal leukoencephalopathy. *Ann Pharmacother.* 2001 Jun;35(6):741–4.

[58] De Luca A, Ammassari A, Pezzotti P, Cinque P, Gasnault J, Berenguer J, et al. Cidofovir in addition to antiretroviral treatment is not effective for AIDS-associated progressive multifocal leukoencephalopathy: a multicohort analysis. *AIDS.* 2008 Sep 12;22(14):1759–67.

[59] Naess H, Glad S, Storstein A, Rinaldo CH, Mørk SJ, Myhr K-M, et al. Progressive multifocal leucoencephalopathy in an immunocompetent patient with favourable outcome. A case report. *BMC Neurol.* 2010;10:32.

[60] Huang SS, Skolasky RL, Dal Pan GJ, Royal W, McArthur JC. Survival prolongation in HIV-associated progressive multifocal leukoencephalopathy treated with alpha-interferon: an observational study. *J Neurovirol.* 1998 Jun;4(3):324–32.

[61] Geschwind MD, Skolasky RI, Royal WS, McArthur JC. The relative contributions of HAART and alpha-interferon for therapy of progressive multifocal leukoencephalopathy in AIDS. *J Neurovirol.* 2001 Aug;7(4):353–7.

[62] Nath A, Venkataramana A, Reich DS, Cortese I, Major EO. Progression of progressive multifocal leukoencephalopathy despite treatment with beta-interferon. *Neurology.* 2006 Jan 10;66(1):149–50.

[63] Przepiorka D, Jaeckle KA, Birdwell RR, Fuller GN, Kumar AJ, Huh YO, et al. Successful treatment of progressive multifocal leukoencephalopathy with low-dose interleukin-2. *Bone Marrow Transplant.* 1997 Dec;20(11):983–7.

[64] Kunschner L, Scott TF. Sustained recovery of progressive multifocal leukoencephalopathy after treatment with IL-2. *Neurology.* 2005 Nov 8;65(9):1510.

[65] Elphick GF, Querbes W, Jordan JA, Gee GV, Eash S, Manley K, et al. The human polyomavirus, JCV, uses serotonin receptors to infect cells. *Science*. 2004 Nov 19;306(5700):1380–3.

[66] Cettomai D, McArthur JC. Mirtazapine use in human immunodeficiency virus-infected patients with progressive multifocal leukoencephalopathy. *Arch Neurol.* 2009 Feb;66(2):255–8.

[67] Kalisch A, Wilhelm M, Erbguth F, Birkmann J. Progressive Multifocal Leukoencephalopathy in Patients with a Hematological Malignancy: Review of Therapeutic Options. *Chemotherapy. 2014* Nov 6;60(1): 47–53.

[68] Marzocchetti A, Tompkins T, Clifford DB, Gandhi RT, Kesari S, Berger JR, et al. Determinants of survival in progressive multifocal leukoencephalopathy. *Neurology.* 2009 Nov 10;73(19):1551–8.

[69] Focosi D, Fazzi R, Montanaro D, Emdin M, Petrini M. Progressive multifocal leukoencephalopathy in a haploidentical stem cell transplant recipient: a clinical, neuroradiological and virological response after treatment with risperidone. *Antiviral Res.* 2007 May;74(2):156–8.

[70] Brickelmaier M, Lugovskoy A, Kartikeyan R, Reviriego-Mendoza MM, Allaire N, Simon K, et al. Identification and characterization of mefloquine efficacy against JC virus in vitro. *Antimicrob Agents Chemother.* 2009 May;53(5):1840–9.

[71] Clifford DB, Nath A, Cinque P, Brew BJ, Zivadinov R, Gorelik L, et al. A study of mefloquine treatment for progressive multifocal leukoencephalopathy: results and exploration of predictors of PML outcomes. *J Neurovirol.* 2013 Aug;19(4):351–8.

[72] Park JH, Ryoo S, Noh HJ, Seo JM, Kang HH, Shin JS, et al. Dual therapy with cidofovir and mirtazapine for progressive multifocal leukoencephalopathy in a sarcoidosis patient. *Case Rep Neurol.* 2011 Sep;3(3):258–62.

[73] Yoshida H, Ohshima K, Toda J, Kusakabe S, Masaie H, Yagi T, et al. Significant improvement following combination treatment with mefloquine and mirtazapine in a patient with progressive multifocal leukoencephalopathy after allogeneic peripheral blood stem cell transplantation. *Int J Hematol.* 2014 Jan;99(1):95–9.

[74] Moenster RP, Jett RA. Mirtazapine and mefloquine therapy for progressive multifocal leukoencephalopathy in a patient infected with human immunodeficiency virus. *Am J Health Syst Pharm.* 2012 Mar 15;69(6):496–8.

[75] Vulliemoz S, Lurati-Ruiz F, Borruat F-X, Delavelle J, Koralnik IJ, Kuntzer T, et al. Favourable outcome of progressive multifocal leucoencephalopathy in two patients with dermatomyositis. *J Neurol Neurosurg Psychiatr.* 2006 Sep;77(9):1079–82.

[76] Thoden J, Potthoff A, Bogner JR, Brockmeyer NH, Esser S, Grabmeier-Pfistershammer K, et al. Therapy and prophylaxis of opportunistic infections in HIV-infected patients: a guideline by the German and Austrian AIDS societies (DAIG/ÖAG) (AWMF 055/066). *Infection.* 2013 Sep;41 Suppl 2:S91–115.

[77] Christensen KLY, Holman RC, Hammett TA, Belay ED, Schonberger LB. Progressive multifocal leukoencephalopathy deaths in the USA, 1979-2005. *Neuroepidemiology.* 2010;35(3):178–84.

[78] Harrison DM, Newsome SD, Skolasky RL, McArthur JC, Nath A. Immune reconstitution is not a prognostic factor in progressive multifocal leukoencephalopathy. *J Neuroimmunol.* 2011 Sep 15;238(1-2):81–6.

[79] García-Suárez J, de Miguel D, Krsnik I, Bañas H, Arribas I, Burgaleta C. Changes in the natural history of progressive multifocal leukoencephalopathy in HIV-negative lymphoproliferative disorders: impact of novel therapies. *Am J Hematol.* 2005 Dec;80(4):271–81.

In: Progressive Multifocal Leukoencephalopathy ISBN: 978-1-63482-889-5
Editor: Denise S. Coleman

Chapter 4

PROGRESSIVE MULTIFOCAL LEUKOENCEPHALOPATHY: RISK FACTORS RELATED TO DRUGS AND MANAGEMENT STRATEGIES

Ana Fernández Pérez and Santiago Piñeiro Conde
Pharmacy Service, University Hospital Lucus Augusti,
Lugo, Spain

ABSTRACT

Progressive multifocal leukoencephalopathy (PML) is a debilitating and frequently fatal central nervous system demyelinating disease caused by JC virus (JCV), for which there is currently no effective treatment. Lytic infection of oligodendrocytes in the brain leads to their eventual destruction and progressive demyelination, resulting in multiple foci of lesions in the white matter of the brain. The recent advent of humanized monoclonal antibody therapy for the treatment of autoimmune inflammatory diseases such as multiple sclerosis and Crohn's disease has also led to an increased risk of PML as a side effect of immunotherapy. We would like to highlight the importance of a correct diagnostic assessment of the viral strain involved in the pathogenesis of PML, and the urgent need to identify possible risk factors and sensitive biomarkers detectable in the early phase of the disease. The study of JCV and the elucidation of the underlying causes of PML are important and active areas of research that may lead to new insights into immune function and host antiviral defense, as well as to potential new therapies. A combined approach with multiple compounds both interfering with different phases of the viral cycle and boosting specific components of the immune system involved in the response to JCV infection should be used.

Progressive Multifocal Leukoencephalopathy and JC Virus

Progressive Multifocal Leukoencephalopathy (PML) is a disease that is anatomopathologically characterized by varying degrees of demyelination in distinct central nervous system sites. It tends to affect the cortical white matter of the parietal and occipital lobes, without accompanying inflammatory changes in cerebrospinal fluid. A triad of symptoms has been described to identify patients suffering from PML, including the rapid deterioration of visual (homonymous hemianopia or cortical blindness), motor and cognitive functions, with motor abnormalities (weakness or hemiparesis) being the most common cause of consultation. PML is considered to be a serious complication of HIV, with some 5-10% of all Acquired Immune Deficiency Syndrome (AIDS) patients developing this illness.[1, 2] It also appears in patients receiving organ or bone marrow transplants, and most recently, in those undergoing immunomodulatory treatment, particularly those containing certain monoclonal antibodies, such as natalizumab, rituximab, infliximab and efalizumab [3].

PML is caused by the Jacob-Creutzfeldt virus (JCV), a polyomavirus that is a member of the Papovaviridae family. Approximately 60 to 80% of the adult population has JC antibodies; however, PML is rarely diagnosed [4]. The primary JC infection typically occurs prior to adolescence with no clinical illness being apparent. The virus tends to cause an asymptomatic infection that is confined to certain tissues. In cases of immunosuppression, it may be reactivated, causing the pathology, most commonly associated with nephropathy and PML.

The JC virus is usually described as strictly neurotrophic; but recently, it has been found to infect other types of cells. It has been detected in amygdaline tissue, suggesting that it may use the respiratory tract as a point of entry, with the tonsils being a potential site of the initial, usually asymptomatic infection [5].

It may remain latent in the tonsil tissue, the stromal tissue of bone marrow, the epithelial cells of the colon and kidneys, etc. It can subsequently infect the peripheral blood lymphocytes that cross the blood-brain barrier during periods of immune deficiency, transporting the virus to the central nervous system [6]. Here, the virus adheres to the infected cells through specific glycoprotein receptors which bind with sialic acid. [7] Serotonin receptor participation is also possible.

Once the virus has entered the cell via endocytosis, its DNA is released and it enters the cell nucleus, since it requires the DNA replication and transcription provided by the growing cell. Finally, the new viruses come together and are released.

Progressive Multifocal Leukoencephalopathy and Drugs

Since the introduction of new biotechnological medications such as monoclonal antibodies and the increasing frequency of immunosuppressive treatments, an increased number of PML cases have been detected. These new cases appear in patients with clinical profiles differing from those of traditionally susceptible patients, such as those suffering from hematopoietic malignancies, those receiving organ and stem cell transplants or those suffering from HIV. [8] Currently, PML associated with the use of natalizumab in patients suffering from multiple sclerosis is the most frequently examined situation, but cases have also been found in patients being treated with other medications, such as those suffering from Crohn's disease under treatment with anti-TNF therapy, patients with systemic lupus erythematosus being treated with efalizumab or patients with lymphoproliferative pathologies or systemic lupus erythematosus taking rituximab.

Not all medications present the same risks for PML and not all of the mechanisms causing this serious complication are understood.

The Food and Drug Administration (FDA) added a "Black Box" alerting to the risk of PML from a large number of medications, a risk that varies greatly depending on the specific medication.

The European Medicines Agency (EMA) has also described the risk for developing PML in their public assessment report (EPAR) in the case in which said information is available at the time of authorization of the medicine or to be updated in upcoming revisions of the document. Neither the FDA nor the EMA have established or stratified the risk of developing PML; they merely provide information.

A classification of the risk of developing PML, originally proposed by Zaheer and Berger in 2012 [9] and subsequently updated by Chahin and Berger in 2014 [10], is presented below.

This classification is based on the known and documented risks and the medicines have been classified based on their risk of causing PML. The classification is intended to serve as a clinical tool for use in decision making processes.

Three categories or classes of medications have been identified, based on their risks of causing PML. They are classified based on the frequency with which PML is detected, the nature of the illness that was being treated, in case the illness itself may have caused a predisposition for developing PML, and the time between the onset of treatment and the development of PML.

The medicines included in the first category present a high risk of developing PML, having an extended period of latency between the onset of treatment and the development of PML. They are used for the treatment of conditions that are not known to cause PML. On the other hand, the medicines classified in category 2 are used in the treatment of pathologies having recognized predispositions for causing PML. The time of PML onset is random and in these cases, there is no period of latency, as observed in the medicines from category 1. The medicines included in the third category are at a low risk for causing PML with only a sporadic number of cases having been found.

Class 1 Therapeutic Agents

Two medications have been identified in this group: natalizumab and efalizumab. Both have been found to clearly increase the risk of developing PML in patients who are not known to have a predisposition for the illness. Furthermore, the latency period between the onset of use of natalizumab or efalizumab and the appearance of PML varies from months to years.

Natalizumab: approved by the EMA for the treatment of relapsing forms of multiple sclerosis (MS) and by the FDA for the treatment of MS and Crohn´s disease.

Natalizumab is a recombinant, humanized form of a murine monoclonal antibody that binds to the α4 subunit of α4β1 and α4β7 integrin. The α4-integrins are expressed on all leukocytes, with the exception neutrophils, as well as hematopoietic progenitor cells, and mediate several homing and adhesive functions. Natalizumab effectively blocks the interaction of α4-

integrins with their cognate receptors. Disruption of these molecular interactions prevents migration of mononuclear leukocytes across the endothelium and into inflamed tissue. Natalizumab may also suppress ongoing inflammatory reactions in diseased tissues by inhibiting α4-expressing leukocytes from binding with its ligands within the extracellular matrix.

In USA, natalizumab was briefly withdrawn for the market in 2005 and was later reintroduced in 2006 under strict surveillance and risk minimization programs.

As of Dec 3, 2014, the overall incidence of PML in natalizumab-treated patients is 3.78 per 1000 patients (95% CI 3.46 to 4.12 per 1000 patients). 77% patients are alive with varying levels of disability. (Biogen US Tysabri Update at website http:// medinfo.biogenidec.com).

Three risk factors related to the development of PML have been identified in patients treated with natalizumab: the presence of anti-JCV antibodies, the duration of treatment with natalizumab (more or less than 24 months) and the use of immunosuppressants prior to the onset of treatment with natalizumab [11, 12].

The risk of PML remains very low (less than 1 in 1000) in patients who had never been exposed to the virus (anti-JCV antibodies negative), irrespective of duration of treatment. The risk is also low in patients who are JCV antibody positive in the first 24 months; in fact, natalizumab-associated PML has not been seen prior to 8n months of therapy and is very rare before 12 months of therapy.

The risk increases significantly after 2 years of use in JCV antibody positive patients, especially in those with history of prior immunosuppressive use [12].

The detection of anti-JCV antibodies via the two-step enzyme immunoassay (ELISA), has been found to be a reliable method of stratifying the risk of PML in patients treated with natalizumab. In fact, this assay has allowed for the documentation of the seroprevalence of anti-JCV antibodies in 50 to 70% of these patients [13]. According to Biogen Idec data collected on the 3rd of December of 2014, 99% of PML patients with available pre-PML samples tested positive for anti-JCV antibodies. The use of antibody levels is a fundamental tool in classifying patients according to risk level.

Prior initiating any treatment with natalizumab, the risk-benefit balance for the patient should be carefully assessed based on his/her individual risk factors for developing PML. A close follow up should be conducted in which the levels of anti-JCV antibodies should be periodically controlled. Efalizumab: a monoclonal antibody originally approved for the treatment of psoriasis. It was withdrawn from the market in USA and Europe because of the risk of serious effects including PML. Efalizumab shares similarities with natalizumab in its mechanism of action: binds specifically to a leukocyte cell surface protein. By preventing this binding, efalizumab may alleviate signs and symptoms of psoriasis by inhibiting several stages in the immunologic cascade.

Given the fact that it is no longer on the market, there is very limited data on risk factors for developing PML in patients taking efalizumab, although research suggests that the duration of treatment may be an important factor [14].

Class 2 Therapeutic Agents

The medications included in this group present a considerably lower risk of causing PML. In fact, in many cases, in this class, PML appears in the context of illnesses that are predisposed to presenting this complication, without the prior use of immunosuppressant treatments. This group includes biological agents such as rituximab, belimumab, brentuximab vedotin, as well as non-biological agents such as mycophenolate mofetil.

Rituximab is a monoclonal antibody approved for treatment of Non-Hodgkin´s Lymphoma, Chronic Lymphocytic Leukemia, Rheumatoid Arthritis, Wegener´s Granulomatosis and Microscopic Polyangiitis. It is also used in other pathologies when scientific evidence justifies its use, even if it is not included in the medication's marketing authorization as is the case with systematic lupus erythematosus, neuromyelitis optica and idiopathic thrombocytopenia purpura, etc. [15].

Rituximab is a chimeric monoclonal antibody that depletes B and pre-B cells that express CD20. Transactivation of JCV in the predominant immature B cells in rituximab-treated patients [16] and reduction of Cd3+ T cells in the cerebral spinal fluid [17] both contribute to the risk of PML.

The risk of developing PML from the use of rituximab is difficult to determine, since this medication tends to be taken by patients suffering from underlying immunological disorders as well as those undergoing immunosuppressant treatments. In fact, there have been no reported cases of PML in patients taking rituximab who did not suffer from illnesses that have known predispositions for PML, such as MS.

While the incidence of PML in rituximab-treated patient is low, the mortality is high with a case fatality rate of 90-100% within 3 months of the last dose of rituximab, a discrepancy that can be explained by the nature of the underlying illness [18].

Mycophenolate Mofetil

Mycophenolate mofetil (MPA) is approved for the prophylaxis of acute transplant rejection in patients receiving allogeneic renal, cardiac or hepatic transplants.

This drug is also used for treatment of several autoimmune disorders [19]. MPA inhibits T and B cells proliferation and impairs immune surveillance for JCV.

MPA-related cases of PML tend to develop without a latency period. They appear in patients having pathologies that may be predisposed to PML or who are being treated with other immunosuppressant drugs [20].

Brentuximab Vedotin

Brentuximab vedotin (BV) is approved for the treatment of refractory Hodgkin´s lymphoma and refractory anaplastic large cell lymphoma. BV is a monoclonal antibody targeting CD30-positive cells, which is conjugated to the cytotoxic agent monomethyl auristatin E. The BV “black box warning” identified potential contributory risk factors as underlying lymphoproliferative disorders, compromised immune systems and multiagent chemotherapy [21].

Belimmab

Belimumab is a humanized antibody approved for the treatment of systemic lupus erythematosus (SLE). It is directed against soluble B-lymphocyte stimulator, an essential growth factor for B-cell maturation and activation.

Patients with SLE are at an increased risk of PML out of proportion to the degree of their immunosuppression. Some have hypothesized that suppression of B cells might prompt proliferation and CNS translocation of infected pre-B lymphocytes, or alternately might have an indirect effect by influencing T-cell control of JCV replication [22].

Class 3 Therapeutic Agents

The medications included in this group are rarely associated with PML, thus their risk level is difficult to determine. As occurs with the class 2 medications, they tend to be used in the treatment of clinical conditions that may have a predisposition for PML and they may even be administered together with other medicines that are associated with a certain risk of developing this complication, therefore accurate data interpretation may be difficult. This class includes agents such as alemtuzumab, TNF-alpha inhibitors, fludarabina, fumaric acid and fingolimod.

Alemtuzumab

Alemtuzumab is approved for treatment of B-cell chronic lymphocytic leukemia (B-CLL) and for MS in USA and only for MS in Europe. Alemtuzumab was withdrawn for the market in Europe for the treatment of B-CLL in 2012.

Alemtuzumab is a humanized monoclonal antibody against D52 expressed primarily on the surface of normal and malignant peripheral blood B and T cell lymphocytes.

It causes the lysis of lymphocytes by binding to CD52, a highly expressed, nonmodulating antigen which is present on the surface of essentially all B and T cell lymphocytes as well as monocytes, thymocytes and macrophages. Although B cells repopulate within 5 to 6 months, T cells deplete for more than 1 year [23].

PML has been reported with alemtuzumab in the background of malignancy or immunosupresion [24, 25]. To date, no reported cases of PML have been seen in the MS cohorts being treated with this agent [24].

TNF-Alpha Inhibitors

TNF-alpha inhibitors include agents such as adalimumab, etanercept, golimumab, certolizumab and infliximab. They are used for the treatment of several autoimmune diseases, rheumatoid arthritis, psoriasis, Crohn's disease and ulcerative colitis.

The common pathway for these agents in the inhibition of tumor necrosis factor-alpha and the resulting decrease in interleukins, specifically IL5 and IL1, and reduction in inflammation and cell recruitment. PML risk with these agents is very small and is confounded by the use of other immunosuppressive agents like metotrexato [14, 26].

Fludarabine

Fludarabine is a chemotherapeutic agent for the treatment of hematologic malignancies. CLL was the most frequent underlying lymphoproliferative disorder that develops PML. It is considered that the immunosuppressive effect of this therapy may cause JCV activation. Another investigation suggests that immunosuppression caused by hematologic malignancies alone may be a factor in the development of PML and fludarabine may act as an additional trigger [27].

Fumaric Acid

Fumaric acid esters are a group of compounds that have been used for the treatment of psoriasis. Dimethylfumarate was approved for the treatment of relapsing forms of MS. These agents exert an immunomodulatory effect through a reduction in the number of T cells.

Case of fumaric acid related PML were reported but occurred either in compounded agents or were confounded by treatment with other immunosuppressive agents.

Manifestation of PML while on dimethylfumarate, with previous monoclonal antibody treatment, gains broader significance. Especially patients treated with natalizumab for two years or longer may wish to discontinue use due to the increasing risk of PML. This sequence of treatments requires careful surveillance [28]. Recently, one case of PML was reported in a patient with MS treated with dimethylfumarate with no current or prior immunosuppressive use.

Fingolimod

Fingolimod is approved for the treatment of relapsing forms of MS. Fingolimod is a sphingosine 1-phosphate (S1P) receptor agonist and it binds with high affinity to S1P receptors, thereby sequestering lymphocytes in the lymph nodes and preventing their egress into the peripheral circulation. Most PML cases observed on fingolimod occurred in patients previously treated with natalizumab.

As dimethylfumarate, the sequence of fingolimod-natalizumab requires careful surveillance.

In 2015, January, the first case of reported PML occurred without prior natalizumab use having been confirmed (information courtesy of Novartis).

Other Class 3 Agents

Several other agents carry a Black Box warning for PML including alkylating agents such as cyclophosphamide, carmustine, dacarbazine; purine analogs such as azathioprine; antimetabolites such as methotrexate; and other immunosuppressants such as cyclosporine and tacrolimus. Few cases of PML have been reported in patients being treated with these agents, and virtually, all cases had an underlying illness predisposing them to PML such as SLE, rheumatoid arthritis and vasculitis or were concurrently treated with other immunosuppressants.

Prevention and Treatment of Progressive Multifocal Leukoencephalopathy

Although a variety of strategies have been published to minimize the risks of developing PML, they are all based mainly on the following aspects: a detailed knowledge of the patient's clinical state including all pharmacological treatments prescribed for the pathology or exposure to medications that may cause PML and the determination of anti-JCV antibodies to determine whether or not the patient is a carrier. Based on these aspects, the medication with the best benefit-risk profile should be carefully selected for the patient.

Chahin and Berger propose a class-specific risk mitigation strategy. PML risk is best studied for class 1 agents, notably natalizumab. As mentioned previously, there are three known risk factors for PML in natalizumab-treated patients; those with one or more of the risk factors for PML are at an increased risk and should be monitored more closely. JCV seronegative patients should undergo repeat determination every 3 to 6 months to monitor for seroconversion. Natalizumab discontinuation should be considered in those patients who are seropositive and have been on treatment for over 1–2 years. In the event that this is not possible or undesirable, patients should be monitored closely both clinically, radiographically, and with JCV antibody titers because early detection of PML is helpful in removal of the agent with plasmapheresis and restoration of normal immune function. Those patients who carry all three risk factors have a very high risk for the development of PML that parallels that of the PML risk with HIV/AIDS prior to the antiretroviral era, and considerations for switching therapy should be made.

Because the risk in class 2 and class 3 agents depends on the underlying disorder and on treatment with other immunosuppressive agents, patients should be assessed and counselled on an individual basis. The risk for PML in these two categories, especially for class 3 drugs, remains small and should be recognized as such. Serologic testing for JCV exposure in classes 2 and 3 agents is not recommended as there is insufficient evidence for its utility in class 2 or 3 agents [10]. Figure 1. Establishing a diagnosis of PML requires the identification of JCV DNA in the cerebral spinal fluid in conjunction with the characteristic neuroimaging findings or the demonstration of the typical histopathological triad, and coupled with the techniques to show the presence of JCV [29]. The fundamental first step in treating confirmed or suspected PML in the setting of an offending agent is discontinuing the treatment and reversing the effects of the drug [20].

The only therapeutic approach that has shown proven clinical efficacy in PML remains the restoration of systemic or local anti-JCV T-cell responses. This restoration can be achieved in patients with acquired immune deficiency syndrome (AIDS) through effective antiretroviral treatment, and in patients with natalizumab-treated multiple sclerosis through natalizumab withdrawal and plasma exchange.

In contrast, there are no effective therapeutic options for patients who are HIV-seronegative with lymphopenia-associated PML [30].

Several agents have been used to treat PML, although these treatments have been based on limited data, and none has proven consistently effective against JCV.

In vitro studies of various compounds with anti-JCV activities showed that only mefloquine, an antimalarial agent, has sufficiently high penetration into the central nervous system.

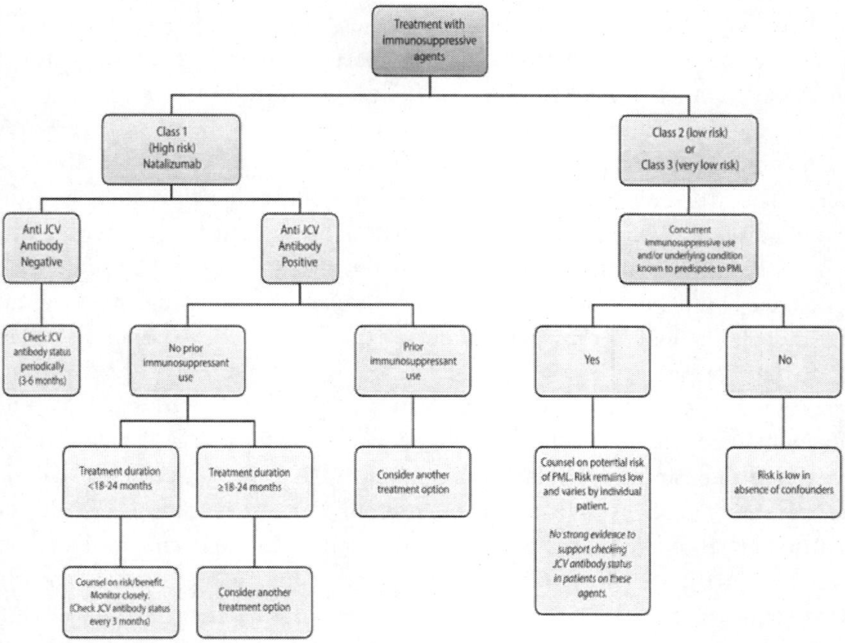

Figure 1. Diagnosis of PML.

Additional experiments demonstrated that mefloquine inhibits the viral infection rates of three JCV isolates: JCV (Mad1), JCV(Mad4), and JCV(M1/SVEDelta). This effect is exerted in three cell types: transformed human glial cells, primary human fetal glial cells, and primary human astrocytes. Mefloquine was also shown to inhibit viral DNA replication when quantitative PCR was used to determine the number of viral copies in cultured cells [29].

The 5-HT2A serotonin receptor has been found to act as a receptor for JCV in glial cells, the use of medications selective for these receptors, such as the antidepressant mirtazapine and antipsychotic risperidone, appears warranted. These classes of medications have been shown to inhibit viral entry into unaffected glial cells.

There have been several case reports on the successful use of mefloquine alone or in combination with mirtazapine in treatment of non-HIV PML.

The use of either of these agents has not been shown to improve outcomes in large prospective studies [31].

The lipid formulation hexadecyloxypropyl-cidofovir (CMX001) has shown activity against JCV in vitro. One PML patient has also been treated successfully with a combination of CMX001 and recombinant human interleukin-7 (rhIL-7), but additional studies are required to confirm the antiviral effect of CMX001 in vivo [30]. No specific antiviral treatment has shown clear clinical efficacy in PML.

The return of immune function is often associated with an entity referred to as immune reconstitution inflammatory syndrome (IRIS). IRIS is a paradoxical worsening of the clinical condition attributed to recovery of the immune system. Although first described in patients with HIV infection with PML and other opportunistic infections, it occurs with other conditions associated with rapid immune recovery, such as following natalizumab withdrawal. PML-IRIS has been observed in 18% of HIV-associated PML cases but appears to be almost invariable based on new or worsening symptoms or magnetic resonance imaging findings with natalizumabassociated PML. Pathological examination of affected tissue reveals an intense perivascular inflammation with CD8+ T cells. PML-IRIS can be associated with significant morbidity and mortality. While no controlled trial regarding treatment has been conducted, preliminary data from both the experience with HIV-associated and natalizumab-associated PML-IRIS suggests that treatment with high-dose intravenous corticosteroids ameliorates the condition. The duration of therapy remains to be determined, but PML-IRIS may last from weeks to months [20].

CONCLUSION

The marketing of new biologically-based medications and the increasingly complex treatments being used for auto-immune diseases have changed the incidence of PML, creating a new profile of patients who may be susceptible to acquiring this serious complication. Physicians should be aware of the risks associated with medications and inherent in patients in order to select the best options, maximizing treatment efficiency and minimizing potential adverse effects. Patients should be adequately informed of the potential risks and benefits associated with their treatment during the decision making process. Patients receiving category 1 treatments should know how to recognize symptoms and signs of PML and they should be carefully controlled, both clinically as well as radiologically.

Publication of the cases of PML associated with new treatments that are available on the market permit physicians to update their knowledge on an on-going basis, a useful tool to assist in this complicated decision-making process.

The study of JCV and the elucidation of the underlying causes of PML are important and active areas of research that may lead to new insights into immune function and host antiviral defense, as well as to potential new therapy.

REFERENCES

[1] Berger J. R., Major E. O. Progressive multifocal leukoencephalopathy. *Semin. Neurol.,* 1999; 19: 193-200.

[2] Berger J. R., Levy R. M., Flomenhoft D., Dobbs M. Predictive factors for prolonged survival in acquired immunodeficiency syndrome-associated progressive multifocal leukoencephalopathy. *Ann. Neurol.,* 1998; 44: 341-349.

[3] Tan C. S., Koralnik I. J. Progressive multifocal leukoencephalopathy and other disorders caused by JC virus: clinical features and pathogenesis. *Lancet Neurol.,* 2010; 9: 425-437.

[4] Khalili K., White M. K., Lublin F., Ferrante P., Berger J. R. Reactivation of JC virus and development of PML in patients with multiple sclerosis. *Neurology,* 2007; 68: 985-990.

[5] Agostini H. T., Jobes D. V., Stoner G. L. Molecular evolution and epidemiology of JC virus. In: *Human polyomaviruses: molecular perspectives. John Wiley and Sons (eds.),* 2001; 491-526.

[6] Sabath B. F., Major E. O. Traffi c of JC virus from sites of initial infection to the brain: the path to progressive multifocal leukoencephalopathy. *J. Infect. Dis.,* 2002; 186 (suppl. 2): S180-86.

[7] Liu C. K., Wei G., et al. Infection of glial cells by the human polyomavirus JC is mediated by an N-linked glycoprotein containing terminal alpha (2-6) linked sialic acids. *J. Virol., 1*998; 72: 4643-9.

[8] Toussirot É., Bereau M. The risk of progressive multifocal leukoencephalopathy under biological agents used in the treatment of chronic inflammatory diseases. *Inflamm. Allergy Drug Targets,* 2014; 13(2):121-7.

[9] Zaheer F., Berger J. R. Treatment related progressive multifocal leukoencephalopathy: current understanding and future steps. *Ther. Adv. Drug Saf.*, 2012; 3:227–239.

[10] Chahin S., Berger J. R. A risk classification for immunosuppressive treatment-associated progressive multifocal leukoencephalopathy. *J. Neurovirol.*, 2014; DOI 10.1007/s13365-014-0303-1.

[11] Fernández O., et al. Consenso espa□nol sobre la utilización de natalizumab (Tysabri®) - 2011. *Neurología,* 2011. doi:10.1016/ j.nrl.2011.09.008.

[12] Sorensen P. S., Bertolotto A., Edan G., Giovannoni G., Gold R., Havrdova E., Kappos L., Kieseier B. C., Montalban X., Olsson T. Risk stratification for progressive multifocal leukoencephalopathy in patients treated with natalizumab. *Mult. Scler.*, 2012; 18:143–152.

[13] Plavina T., Subramanyam M., Bloomgren G., Richman S., Pace A., Lee S., Schlain B., Campagnolo D., Belachew S., Ticho B. Anti-JCV antibody levels in serum or plasma further define risk of natalizumab-associated PML. *Ann. Neurol.*, 2014; 76(6):802-12.

[14] Kothary N., Diak I. L., Brinker A., Bezabeh S., Avigan M., Dal Pan G. Progressive multifocal leukoencephalopathy associated with efalizumab use in psoriasis patients. *J. Am. Acad. Dermatol.*, 2011; 65:546–551.

[15] I. Danés, A. Agustí, A. Vallano, C. Alerany, J. Mrtínez, J. A. Bosch, A. Ferrer, L. Gratacós, A. Pérez, M. Olmo, S. M. Cano Marron, A. Valderrama, X. Bonafont. Outcomes of off-label drug uses in hospitals: a multicentric prospective study. *Eur. J. Clin. Pharmacol.*, 2014; 70:1385–1393.

[16] Leandro M. J., Cambridge G., Ehrenstein M. R., Edwards J. C. Reconstitution of peripheral blood B cells after depletion with rituximab in patients with rheumatoid arthritis. *Arthritis Rheum.*, 2006; 54:613–620.

[17] Cross A. H., Stark J. L., Lauber J., Ramsbottom M. J., Lyons J. A. Rituximab reduces B cells and T cells in cerebrospinal fluid of multiple sclerosis patients. *J. Neuroimmunol.*, 2006; 180:63–70.

[18] Carson K. R., Evens A. M., Richey E. A., Habermann T. M., Focosi D., Seymour J. F., Laubach J., Bawn S. D., Gordon L. I., Winter J. N., Furman R. R., Vose J. M., Zelenetz A. D., Mamtani R., Raisch D. W., Dorshimer G. W., Rosen S. T., Muro K., Gottardi-Littell N. R., Talley R. L., Sartor O., Green D., Major E. O., Bennett C. L. Progressive multifocal leukoencephalopathy after rituximab therapy in HIV-negative patients: a report of 57 cases from the Research on Adverse Drug Events and Reports project. *Blood,* 2009; 113:4834–4840.

[19] Villarroel M. C., Hidalgo M., Jimeno A. Mycophenolate mofetil: an update. *Drugs Today (Barc),* 2009; 45:521–532.

[20] Berger J. R. Progressive multifocal leukoencephalopathy and newe rbiological agents. *Drug Saf.,* 2010; 33:969–983.

[21] Carson K. R. et al. Progressive multifocal leukoencephalopathy associated with brentuximab vedotin therapy: a report of 5 cases from the Southern Network of Adverse Reactions (SONAR) project. *Cancer,* 2014; 120(16): 2464-71.

[22] Fredericks C., Kvam K., Bear J., Crabtree G., Josephson S. A case of progressive multifocal leukoencephalopathy in a lupus patient treated with belimumab. *Lupus,* 2014; 23:711-713.

[23] Wingerchuk D. M., Carter J. L. Multiple Sclerosis: Current and Emerging Disease-Modifying Therapies and Treatment Strategies. *Mayo Vin. Pro.,* 2014; 89(2): 225-240.

[24] Isidoro L., Pires P., Rito L., Cordeiro G. Progressive multifocal leukoencephalopathy in a patient with chronic lymphocytic leukaemia treated with alemtuzumab. *BMJ Case Rep.,* 2014. doi:10.1136/bcr-2013-201781.

[25] Piccinni C., Sacripanti C., Poluzzi E., Motola D., Magro L., Moretti U., Conforti A., Montanaro M. Stronger association of drug-induced progressive multifocal leukoencephalopathy (PML) with biological immunomodulating agents. *Eur. J. Clin. Pharmacol.*, 2010; 66:199–206.

[26] Kumar D., Bouldin T. W., Berger R. G. A case of progressive multifocal leukoencephalopathy in a patient treated with infliximab. *Arthritis Rheum.*, 2010; 62:3191–3195.

[27] Lejniece S., Murovska M., Chapenko S., Breiksa B., Jaunmuktane Z., Feldmane L., Ziedina I., Gomez-Roman J., Garcia-Cabeza M., Lejnieks A. Progressive multifocal leukoencephalopathy following fludarabine treatment in a chronic lymphocytic leukemia patient. *Exp. Oncol.*, 2011: 33:239–241.

[28] Stoppe M., Thomä E., Liebert U. G., Major E. O., Hoffmann K. T., claben J., Bergh F. T. Cerebellar manifestation of PML under fumarate and after efalizumab treatment of psoriasis. *J. Neurol.*, 2014; 261:1021–1024.

[29] Garrote et al. Long-term survival in a patient with progressive multifocal leukoencephalopathy after therapy with rituximab, fludarabine and cyclophosphamide for chronic lymphocytic leukemia. *Experimental Hematology and Oncology,* 2015; 4:8.

[30] Gasnault J. et al. Efficacy of Recombinant Human Interleukin 7 in a Patient With Severe Lymphopenia-Related Progressive Multifocal Leukoencephalopathy. *Open Forum Infect. Dis.*, 2014; 1(2):ofu74.

[31] Epperla N., Medina-Flores R., Mazza J. J., Yale S. H. Mirtazapine and Mefloquine Therapy for Non–AIDSRelated Progressive Multifocal Leukoencephalopathy. *WMJ*, 2014; 113(6):242-5.

In: Progressive Multifocal Leukoencephalopathy ISBN: 978-1-63482-889-5
Editor: Denise S. Coleman

Chapter 5

RISK OF IMMUNE RECONSTITUTION INFLAMMATORY SYNDROME (IRIS) IN NATALIZUMAB-ASSOCIATED PML

Alberto Calvi**, *Milena Alessandra De Riz, Anna Pietroboni, Daniela Galimberti and Elio Scarpini

Neurology Unit, Dept. of Pathophysiology and Transplantation,
University of Milan, Fondazione Ca' Granda,
IRCCS Ospedale Policlinico, Milan, Italy

ABSTRACT

The term "Immune reconstitution inflammatory syndrome" (IRIS) was originally introduced to describe the phenomenon of paradoxical clinical deterioration in HIV-infected patients despite the successful virological and immunological recovery after treatment with antiretroviral therapy.

This condition has actually been described even in the central nervous system (CNS) when immunosuppressed patients experience an opportunistic infection, as a result of an aberrant response of the immune function. Since new immunosuppressant therapies for autoimmune diseases or graft rejection in transplanted patients have been established,

* Phone: +390255033847, Fax: +390255036580, E-mail: albicalvi@libero.it.

IRIS has become much more frequent, as a consequence of sudden immunosuppressive drug removal.

In Natalizumab treated multiple sclerosis (MS) patients, there is a well known risk of developing progressive multifocal encephalopathy (PML), a rare demyelinating disease of the subcortical white matter, requiring the reactivation of latent JCV reservoirs and the subsequent invasion of the CNS. PML typically presents with subacute neurological symptoms that mainly affect cognitive functions, with a progressive course sometimes leading to severe neurological deficits. When PML takes place the standard treatment is plasma exchange (PLEX) or immunoabsorption (IA). The drug removal from bloodstream restores lymphocyte trafficking into the CNS, leading to a massive infiltration into PML lesions.

Evidence from literature describes in nearly all cases of Natalizumab-associated PML the occurrence of IRIS, presenting as a subacute progression and exacerbation of earlier symptoms of PML within days to a few weeks after PLEX. PML-IRIS is the consequence of an enhanced immune response to disease-specific antigens, likely leading to an overproduction of inflammatory mediators.

This condition is differentiated in early or late PML-IRIS by the time course relative to PLEX/IA and contrast enhancement at the brain MRI. There is a variety of patterns of clinical presentation and evolution, ranging from asymptomatic to catastrophic.

The two major factors which contribute to the severity of IRIS are the degree of immune suppression and the rapidity of immune recovery. It has become routine so far to observe that a strong reactivation of the disease, in terms of inflammatory response, is a risk after the suspension of Natalizumab therapy in MS patients. The scientific community is now trying to differentiate the classical IRIS, typically occurring in the setting of PML, from the typical MS rebounds following Natalizumab suspension. Reports of outcomes after discontinuation of therapy suggested an eventual return of disease activity to pretreatment levels in terms of the degree of inflammatory response, which eventually increases with duration of therapy interruption.

In this chapter, we will focus on epidemiology, pathogenesis and treatment of IRIS with particular attention to cases following Natalizumab-associated PML.

1. Introduction to IRIS

Inflammation reflects the physiological response to the presence of infectious antigens, as a consequence of immune natural and adaptive response. In the immunocompetent host, after an incubation period, the extent of inflammation declines progressively as the infectious agent is controlled by the immunological response. However, it is possible to observe a disproportion of the two players, the infectious agent trying to overwhelm the response of immune cells, resulting in excessive inflammation. This scenario is frequent when a condition of immunodepression is present: host inflammation in response to infectious agents is impaired, therefore, in the case of reemerging immunocompetence, an increase of "paradoxical" inflammatory response may develop [1]. This condition resembles a recently acquired acute disease, an uncommon pathophysiologic mechanism arising from the exaggerated immunological response, called Immune Restoration Inflammatory Syndrome (IRIS). The common denominator in this condition, which can develop during a variety of different infections, is a robust immune response that is detrimental to the host.

There has not been a consensus definition of IRIS in literature so far, and many synonyms have been introduced in different pathological conditions, such as Immune Recovery Syndrome, Immune Reconstitution Disease, Immune Reconstitution Syndrome, Immune Restoration Disease, Immune Rebound Illness, Steroid-Withdrawal Disease, Immuno-restitution Disease, Immune Response Reactions. However this condition could be described by the predisposing factors, the clinical manifestations, the therapeutic requirements and the distinct immunopathologic features.

IRIS may be targeted at viable infective antigens, dead or dying infective antigens, host antigens, tumor antigens and other antigens, giving rise to a heterogeneous range of clinical manifestations. This condition may develop in different settings, both in the immunocompetent and the immunodeficient individual.

In the setting of cellular immunodeficiency the typical presentation of IRIS follows the introduction of antiretroviral treatment (ART) of HIV infection, as an unexpected and atypical inflammatory response, occurring predominantly in the condition of previous underlying severe immunosuppression. It is nowadays a common complication, as the increasing and widespread use of ART, consisting of clinical deterioration in the first weeks to months after initiation of therapy, though IRIS can occur as late as 2 years after ART initiation [2]. The incidence of IRIS among people starting ART seems quite frequent (16.1% of individuals in a combined meta-analysis by Müller et al), although variable depending on the different AIDS-defining illness, and higher rates with inversely lowering CD4 cell count at baseline and rapid decline in viral load [3]. Overall mortality is reported to be in the range of 0-15%, considering that IRIS affecting CNS has a particularly high value and represents the most severe form of the syndrome.

In this condition two distinct temporal patterns of disease have been described. "*Paradoxical IRIS*", occurring in the setting of a pre-existing and recognized opportunistic infection for which treatment is under way with beneficial response and reduction of viremia, consists of a clinical acute worsening following the initiation of ART. The second manifestation is marked by the occurrence of a previously not diagnosed opportunistic infection, characterized by an unexpected acute course and a pronounced inflammatory component towards viable pathogens, while starting ART, the so called "*Unmasking IRIS*". The latter condition should be differentiated by an ART associated opportunistic infection, which progresses with a typical clinical course without the atypical features of IRIS. A wide range of pathologies have been recognized in HIV-associated IRIS, including mycobacterial infections, criptococcal meningitis, herpes zoster, cytomegalovirus retinitis, Kaposi's sarcoma, non-Hodgkin lymphoma and progressive multifocal leukoencephalopathy [4-6]. IRIS in HIV patients under ART may develop without an underlying infection, probably due to T cell response directed against the viral reservoirs, especially in the CNS, where it is possible that the inflammatory reaction is driven toward the brain tissue itself. The latter phenomenon is responsible of atypical forms of acute encephalitis.

Finally, IRIS during ART can also develop as progression of proliferative disease in patients with cancer [7] or as an exacerbation of autoimmune diseases [8].

It is to mention that standardized diagnostic test are not available for IRIS, still there are consensus case definitions, for tubercolosis-associated subtype, provided by the International Network for the Study of HIV-associated IRIS [4] helping clinicians to support the suspect of this pathology, after the exclusion of all the other conditions or the unsuccessful treatment of other diseases.

Considering the immunocompetent host, under specific infections, such as multibacillary 'lepromatous' leprosy and disseminated tubercolosis, the occurrence of IRIS is the result of the effective antimicrobial treatment, as it allows the immune system to react with a potent inflammatory response. In the setting of disseminated TBC under tubercolostatic treatment, the shift from negative to positive skin reaction is one of the expression of restoration of immunity typical of IRIS. Furthermore, the occurrence of cerebral tubercoloma may result in a fatal outcome as a result of excessive inflammation. Other examples of inflammatory syndromes associated with immune restoration in the immunocompetent host include hypersensitivity reactions occurring after initiation of antimicrobial therapy for syphilis (the "Jarisch-Herxheimer reaction") [9], bacterial meningitis or antibiotic-induced endotoxin release in sepsis [10].

Other conditions of immunodepression with rapid restoration of immune function have been described related to subsequent IRIS, such as hematopoietic reconstitution after high dose cytostatic chemotherapy in patients with hematologic malignancies, or in transplant recipients after reduction in immunosuppressive therapy often simultaneously with treatment for an opportunistic infection [11].

Recently, new biological therapies for autoimmune diseases resulted in susceptibility to opportunistic infections with an increasing incidence rate of IRIS as major complication, following the withdrawal of the drugs. In clinical setting, this condition is difficult to solve, as the decision to stop immune-modulatory therapies with the aim to allow the immune-cells to fight the opportunistic infection could instead determine a re-activation of the underlying autoimmune disease.

2. IRIS in Natalizumab-Associated PML

Progressive multifocal leukoencephalopathy (PML) is a demyelinating disease caused by infection of the CNS by John Cunningham virus (JCV) occurring in the context of immunosuppression. PML was considered a rare disease, observed in the severely immunosuppressed patients, such as in hematological malignancies and organ transplant recipients, but since HIV epidemic, the prevalence is growing, with 5% of AIDS patients experiencing this condition [12]. Furthermore, PML has emerged as a major complication of immunomodulatory medications for autoimmune diseases, such as natalizumab for Multiple Sclerosis (MS) and Crohn's disease, rituximab for lupus and efalizumab for psoriasis. Therefore, PML occur as a result of the reactivation of latent JCV in peripheral reservoirs, that then invades the CNS.

JCV is a human DNA polyomavirus, causing an asymptomatic primary infection with subsequent quiescence of the virus predominantly in kidney, bone marrow and lymphoid tissue cells but even in neurons and glial cells, as demonstrated by the wide expression of the cellular receptors (an N-linked glycoprotein and 5-HT_{2A} serotoninergic receptor). During immunosuppression, the secondary infection expresses with PML through reactivation of JCV in the CNS and massive lytic infection of oligodendrocytes. The analysis of viral genome has revealed that multiple rearrangements are necessary for the reactivation of the virus which causes PML and that they probably occur during immunosuppression [13]. The cellular immune response is necessary for prevention of viral reactivation and it seems that CD8 cytotoxic T lymphocytes are the main responsible for the elimination of the virus [14].

The reported seroprevalence of JCV varies throughout the literature, ranging between 50 to 90% in recent studies [15].

PML is characterized by a wide variety of subacute neurological deficits, associated with areas of demyelination in the brain, including muscle weakness, sensory deficits, hemianopsia, coordination and gait difficulties. However, the typical picture regards mainly cognitive dysfunctions, such as aphasia, apraxia and subcortical dementia. Involvement of the optic nerves or the spinal cord is unusual, whereas presentation with seizures are more typical of grey matter lesions.

The typical white matter lesions are detected by CT scan, showing hypodense or patchy areas, and more precisely with MRI with widespread asymmetrical hypointense lesions on T1-weighted and hyperintensity on T2-weighted and fluid-attenuated inversion recovery sequences [16]. The lesions are localized more commonly in the parieto-occipital lobes, posterior fossa and, more rarely in the brainstem [17]. Furthermore, PML lesions can be found even in grey matter structures, such as the basal ganglia or the thalamus, in which there are myelinated fibers. It is not common to detect contrast enhancement or mass effect as initial presentation of PML.

The histological finding of PML is a productive, lytic infection of oligodendrocytes and astrocytes along with reactive gliosis in the absence of inflammation, leading to multiple areas of demyelination [18]. Lesions are mainly localized in subcortical white matter, involving arcuate fibers, that enlarge during progression of the disease.

Detection of JCV DNA in the cerebrospinal fluid (CSF) by PCR, together with the typical imaging features, are required for the diagnosis of "definite PML", based on the consensus statement from the American Academy of Neurology [19]. Nevertheless, there are controversial cases where JCV positivity in the CSF is not found, probably due to the occurrence of false negative test [20].

The disease course is usually progressive, leading to neurological deficits or even death, depending on different factors. In HIV-positive patients, a higher CD4+ T-cell count and contrast enhancement on radiographic imaging were associated with longer-term survival [21]. Furthermore, in natalizumab-associated PML a higher load of JCV copies is associated with worse course of the disease and increased mortality [22].

Treatment of PML is directed at favoring the restoration of adaptive immune response in order to suppress viral replication. Consequently, in HIV patients, the continuation of antiretroviral therapy is detrimental. Trials with cidofovir or cytarabine have not proved efficacy in the reduction of mortality or the residual PML-related disability [23-24]. In addition mefloquine was found to have activity against JCV in vitro [25], with relatively good outcome in HIV patient also receiving antiretroviral therapy, then it is difficult to predict its real positive effect. Finally, mirtazapine has been considered for the action against JCV serotonin receptors, however no convincing evidence in vivo has been provided [26].

Natalizumab-associated PML was described shortly after the drug's approval in 2005, as a major complication in MS treatment.

Natalizumab is a monoclonal humanized antibody targeting the α-4 subunit of the integrin adhesion molecule on T lymphocytes (CD49d), favoring the blockade of cell-trafficking across the blood–brain barrier. The effect on lymphocytes is employed to reduce the inflammation of the CNS, which is considered the main pathogenic mechanism in MS.

As of November 2014, more than 500 cases of PML have been reported, in a population of more than 13000 MS patients treated with Natalizumab [27]. The overall incidence of natalizumab-associated PML is approximately 3.72 per 1000 patients.

Established risk factors for development of natalizumab-associated PML include the presence of anti–JCV antibodies in serum or plasma, the use of immunosuppressants (IS) prior to natalizumab treatment and duration of natalizumab treatment beyond 2 years. The lowest risk of developing PML is in the subgroup of patients who tested negative for anti-JCV status, with an estimated PML risk of 1 per 10000 as demonstrated by data from post-marketing sources and the large prospective study STRATIFY-2 [28]. In patients who are anti-JCV antibody positive, PML risk is stratified based on prior IS use and treatment duration. The overall incidence of PML in anti-JCV antibody–positive patients with no prior immunosuppressant use remains <1 per 1,000 patients during the first 2 years of natalizumab treatment. According to recent literature, the duration of natalizumab exposure at PML diagnosis is around 40 months, while nearly 30% of patients had prior IS use [29].

A definite diagnosis of PML is made upon the already cited diagnostic criteria in a patient under natalizumab treatment, but in the absence of clinical symptoms, with MRI suggestive of PML and JCV detection in the CSF, the condition is classified as “probable PML”. This fact outlines the importance of MRI monitoring in natalizumab-treated patients for detecting PML before clinical symptoms occur.

The mortality of natalizumab-associated PML is approximately 25 %, a significantly greater survival rate than in other disease populations, as of recent reports [30].

Treatment of natalizumab-associated PML is based on plasma exchange (PLEX) or immunoabsorbtion (IA), favoring fast drug removal from bloodstream and reconstitution of immune response against the virus. Better outcomes are observed with early diagnosis of Natalizumab-associated PML, drug discontinuation, and plasma exchange initiation. Among the survivor cohort of natalizumab-associated PML, most are left moderately to severely disabled [31].

The majority of patients with natalizumab-associated PML also experience PML-IRIS, presenting as a subacute progression and exacerbation of earlier symptoms of PML within days to a few weeks after PLEX. IRIS may develop within days or up to 2 months following the withdrawal of natalizumab. This condition is differentiated by the time course and clinical pattern, as well as for the imaging MRI features.

In comparison to PML-IRIS in HIV-infected patients, natalizumab-treated patients develop IRIS more frequently, and the IRIS is much more severe [2]. This is consistent with an intact systemic immune system in the natalizumab-treated patients, which provides a rapid influx of lymphocytes from blood to brain, once the Natalizumab is removed.

The fact that cessation of Natalizumab alone, in patients not experiencing any kind of infection, can cause an immunological rebound with IRIS is to consider in the 3 months after cessation of the therapy. However, any clinical deterioration in MS patients after Natalizumab cessation may be considered a relapse of the disease and in the case of pre-treatment high activity of disease (i.e. high value of annualized relapse ratio or high MRI lesion load) the successive immune reactivation is expected to be responsible for a strong inflammatory rebound sometimes mimicking IRIS.

3. Etiology and Pathogenesis

The immunopathogenesis of IRIS remains unclear but it is currently intensely investigated, with interesting discoveries helping to individuate risk factors and the mechanisms favoring this condition.

A verified assumption is that the degree of immune suppression and the rapidity of immune recovery are the two major factors that drive the development of IRIS. This is clear in the setting of HIV infection, as previously described, where the low CD4+ T cells count at baseline and a rapid decline in viral load are associated with a worse outcome [3].

It is important to make considerations about IRIS in the setting of HIV infection, because some evidences of the pathologic mechanisms have been already provided since the identification of this pathological entity. In this condition the innate and adaptive immune responses to dead or alive pathogens lead to the release of cytokines and chemokines, which may differ depending on the type of pathogen. The effects of the cytokines and chemokines produced may include enhancement of Th1 responses (Interleukin-18, Interferon-γ), recruitment of T cells and NK cells to sites of inflammation (Chemokine CXCL-10) and production of inflammatory molecules such as C-reactive protein (Iinterleukin-6) [32]. Recent studies point out that IRIS is considered to be a predominantly CD4-mediated phenomenon as demonstrated by higher frequencies of activated CD4+ cells compared with patients who do not develop IRIS, in the absence of adequate T regulatory cells (T reg) control, with a potential contribution of homeostatic signals [33]. Moreover, HIV-IRIS patients also have increased interferon-gamma (IFNγ) expression and PD-1 expression on T cells (a marker of T cell exhaustion) prior to ART initiation as compared with non-IRIS HIV patients. Host genetic factors may also regulate the robustness of the immune response and hence the development of IRIS, but these factors need to be further studied [34].

Natalizumab-associated PML is the result of re-activation of latent JCV mainly in the oligodendrocytes, producing a lytic infection, with the result of an infective white matter disease of the CNS. It is not well understood which biological factors contribute to the facilitation of this mechanism, but the etiology is probably connected with impaired CNS immune surveillance. For example, in Natalizumab-treated MS patients specific subsets of immune cells (CD4+ and CD8+ T cells, CD19+ B cells, and CD138+ plasma cells) decrease in the CSF during the course of the treatment [35]. This condition, characterized by a general decrease of adaptive immune control, could be the starting point for the perpetuation of viral replication.

In addition to underlying depressed or altered immune function, viral determinants may also increase PML risk and/or disease severity. Genetic studies of viral sequences in PML patients found several mutations in the host cell receptor binding domain of the viral capsid protein (VP1) and in the non-coding control region (NCCR) [36]. These rearrangements, which probably occur during immune suppression, are necessary for the reactivation of JCV that causes PML. This fact partially justifies the low incidence rate of this complication in MS patients treated with natalizumab.

After JCV infection has reemerged in PML patients, the host response is mediated by the cellular immunity. The increased JCV specific antibody titer is not associated to suppression of PML, therefore the humoral immune response alone is not sufficient, even though an intrathecal synthesis of IgG antibodies specific for JCV peptides is found in the majority of patients [37]. CD4+ T cell restricted to the virus are mostly implicated in the response to JCV re-activation, as that they are found in the blood of patients surviving PML and the number of these cells correlates with JCV clearance from the CSF [38]. The importance of CD4+ T cells in the cellular immune response to JCV infection is that initiation and perpetuation of antigen-specific CD8+ T-cell responses may require the help of CD4+ T cells, supplied in the form of cytokines and other inflammatory mediators. As a result, CD8+ cytotoxic T lymphocytes are the main effectors cells, recognizing the epitopes of viral proteins presented on the class I HLA molecules of the infected cells with subsequent elimination and reduction of viral spread. Furthermore, JCV-specific CD8+ T cells are detectable in the peripheral blood of PML patients, and their presence is associated with a more favorable clinical outcome [39].

From a pathological point of view, in PML-IRIS biopsies histology reveals strikingly pronounced inflammation and low numbers of virally infected cells. Moreover, inflammation is even more pronounced than in HIV PML-IRIS, probably because of the effectively reconstituted immune system (and in MS patients otherwise intact) after the withdrawal of Natalizumab. The major inflammatory cells found in PML lesions belong to the CD8+ subset, but even the abundance of plasma cells is remarkable [40]. This finding suggest to reconsider the role of B cells in the pathogenesis of PML-IRIS, together with the observation that Natalizumab treatment increases circulating pre-B and B-cells and that these cells could carry JCV into the CNS [41].

Several studies demonstrate that subclinical JCV reactivation (measured in blood and CSF) is a frequent finding in Natalizumab treated patients and it may depend, at least in part, on the duration of drug exposure [42]. As previously described, higher JC viral load is detected in circulating progenitor CD34+ cells and monocytes compared to other circulating mononuclear cell subpopulations. This is in line with the hypothesis that in Natalizumab-treated patients the virus enters the circulation from hematopoietic latency sites. However, this mechanism is not supported by the fact that Natalizumab prevents cell diapedesis, consequently it is not known how JCV may enter the

CNS. Conceivably, reactivation of latent JCV within the CNS, in the condition of reduced immune surveillance, could be the possible etiological mechanism involved in Natalizumab-associated PML.

Since it has been observed viremia without positive antibody status to JCV in Natalizumab-treated MS patients [43], it is difficult to predict the course and the possible evolution of PML by evaluating immune response to JCV.

Considering PML pathology from an immunological point of view, the presence of Th2 response may play a role in PML development or progression, whereas Th1 cellular response against the virus may be of paramount importance in controlling clinically evident disease. This consideration is supported by the finding of highly prevalent anti-JCV memory and effector T-cell response in Natalizumab-treated MS patients.

One of the challenging problems in IRIS associated to immunosuppressive therapy is that the consequence of the withdrawal of the drug is a rebound of the underlying autoimmune disease.

In MS, Natalizumab function is to block trafficking of lymphocytes into the CNS, as previously described. When PML is suspected, the first step is to stop Natalizumab, trying to facilitate the restoration of physiological immune response and surveillance against microbial agents in the CNS. Nevertheless, in MS patients, this condition means to expose CNS to the risk of autoimmune attack by the restored trafficking of the immune cells, with a massive inflammatory reaction at the site of PML lesions.

4. Clinical and Diagnostic Remarks

IRIS is a frequent complication in patients experiencing Natalizumab-associated PML, occurring in the vast majority of cases, after the regular course of PLEX.

The clinical presentation of IRIS in Natalizumab-associated PML is depicted by a progression or re-acutization of symptoms of PML. This condition has been classified as follows according to the severity of the clinical state [44]:

1. Asymptomatic IRIS: condition not detected by clinical examination, but exclusively by MRI appearance of contrast enhancement;
2. Symptomatic IRIS: objective deterioration of neurological functions accompanied by modification of MRI pattern;

3. Catastrophic IRIS: severe neurologic decline, in the extreme case presenting with coma, associated with signs of brain oedema/herniation at MRI.

This is not a strict classification, as it is often difficult to establish that the clinical condition registered is not evolving during time; in addition, there are few prognostic markers.

The distribution of the clinical patterns at presentation is not fully characterized, but, according to clinical reports and retrospective studies, the majority of patients belong to the second class, showing some symptoms at PML diagnosis. Therefore, it is possible that the re-acutization of IRIS could occur with the same clinical pattern, reasonably with symptomatic patients in the majority of cases. IRIS is suspected to be a risk factor for seizures, an atypical presentation in natalizumab-associated PML cases, considering that classic PML is largely recognized as a white matter process.

Recently, more attention has been given to asymptomatic cases of PML, which have been reported with increasing frequency [29]. Considering that, in Natalizumab-treated patients, MRI is the main tool to monitor the adverse effect of therapy, especially in patients with JCV antibodies positivity, clinicians should be aware that there is a possibility to diagnose PML in the absence of symptoms.

In addition, it is possible to make a radiological classification of PML based on the location of the lesions and on the different imaging patterns at brain MRI. PML lesions are distinguished in unilobar, when confined to one lobe, multilobar, when they are involving two or more contiguous lobes, or widespread, when they affect both hemispheres.

Common MRI features of PML have been widely defined [45]: the typical lesions are large, confluent, and subcortical, thereby involving U-fibers, with a low signal on T1-weighed images and a high signal on T2-weighed and diffusion images. The border is sharp toward the grey matter and ill defined toward the white matter. Additionally, in the majority of cases punctate T2 hyperintensities in the vicinity of PML lesions were observed, with contrast enhancement.

Typically a single white matter lesion is more than 3 cm wide or multiple asymmetric lesions are present, becoming confluent and enlarged as disease progresses, usually without mass effect. Finally, T1-hyperintense signals were found during and after the IRIS phase of PML and could therefore help differentiate PML from PML-IRIS. From a diagnostic point of view, neuroradiological support is essential to formulate a diagnosis of PML and in differentiating the occurrence of an immune reconstitution syndrome, as previously described. The evidence of new inflammatory activity at brain MRI, is one of the cardinal point to support the suspect of PML-IRIS. This represents the main differential diagnostic finding from the classic PML presentation: the evidence of contrast-enhancing lesions at previously reported PML sites or elsewhere in the CNS, which correspond to the immune reconstitution and the subsequent inflammation.

However, recently published case reports show that it is possible, retrospectively, to find some evidence of inflammation at brain MRI, even before Natalizumab cessation in certain type of Natalizumab-associated PML [46]. These cases are referred as "*early PML-IRIS*", because they are more probably followed by a rapidly evolving IRIS just after PLEX, in the range of 3 weeks [47]. A recent study reported the association of hyperintense cortical signal (HCS) on precontrast T1-weighted MR images with higher frequency in IRIS patients [48]. However, HCS is a sign of cortical laminar necrosis, not specific for identifying IRIS.

Considering the detection of JCV by PCR in the cerebrospinal fluid of PML-IRIS patients, there are controversial data, as viral replication might be undetected or, on the contrary, increased viral load is recorded [49].

One of the big challenges for the physician is to predict the clinical course depending on the clinical features and the presentation of the syndrome, as soon as PML has been diagnosed. However, the situation is controversial in literature. On one hand, there is evidence that early PML-IRIS is associated with worse outcome, both in terms of follow-up EDSS and mortality [47]. On the other hand, a shorter time from symptom onset to PML diagnosis (the early forms), and localized disease on MRI at diagnosis have been associated with improved survival [50].

Asymptomatic cases at PML diagnosis were more commonly associated with a favorable pattern at MRI imaging, such as that of unilobar lesions, by higher survival rates and less functional disability at follow-up [29].

A recently published report provided a large-scale analysis of predictors of survival and functional outcomes in the population of patients affected by Natalizumab-associated PML [30]. Survival rate is quite high, with more than two thirds of patients observed more than one year after PML diagnosis. Among survivors, younger age at diagnosis, lower fluid JCV viral load and less extensive disease on MRI proved to be prognostic markers of better functional outcome in terms of Expanded Disability Status Scale (EDSS) and Karnofsky Peroformance Scale (KPS) scores at follow-up. Moreover, it seems that less functional disability pre-PML is associated with a better prognosis at diagnosis and in the subsequent months. However, as reported by recent case reports, even in severe cases of PML-IRIS at diagnosis, requiring intensive care support, the outcome at follow-up may be satisfactory [51]. These data reflect the heterogeneity of the syndrome and the fact that there are yet unknown environmental or genetic factors playing a role in the development of IRIS.

The observation that there are big differences in terms of clinical patterns in PML and related PML-IRIS is provided by all the described data; there is a possibility that the pathological entity might correspond to two different clinical presentations. One form, previously cited as the "early PML-IRIS", which is rapidly progressive, evolving in a time course of months, and another one, with a delayed progression or even late clinical presentation (as for example asymptomatic PML cases manifesting symptoms after months from the radiological diagnosis). This may be due to yet unknown differences in host or viral attributes that may contribute to these observations. Moreover, the differences of the two clinical groups are the result of distinct pathophysiological mechanisms, in terms of a stronger and faster immune response in the "early PML-IRIS". These considerations support the notion that there are common aspects in HIV-infected patients, as they can develop a simultaneous PML-IRIS just following the initiation of ART, or other already diagnosed PML patients may develop in a second time IRIS.

Considering the role of the clinician in front of a deterioration of the clinical condition in MS patients treated with Natalizumab, the caveat is the differential diagnosis between PML, simultaneous PML-IRIS or MS exacerbation. In fact, natalizumab suspension has been associated with a significant disease re-activation within 6 months, often presenting with severe clinical and radiological manifestations, especially in patients with high disease activity before initiating the treatment [52]. Although there are differences in the MRI imaging patterns of the considered different conditions, it is a clinical good practice rule to consider any new clinical or radiological activity in a MS patient undergoing Natalizumab as a possible expression of PML, especially in the condition of JCV antibodies seropositivity.

5. Treatment Options

Treatment for Natalizumab-associated PML is based on the suspension of the drug activity, obtained by removing it by blood with plasma exchange. PLEX is effective in accelerating the clearance of Natalizumab, with a desaturation of less than 50% of alfa4-integrin receptors sensibly faster than without any intervention, which is realized in approximately 2 weeks [53]. Current recommendation is to perform 5 sessions of plasmapheresis, which help to reach the target of reducing the drug concentration below 1 µg/mL, the cut-off to observe the desaturation of drug receptors. However, given that half-life of natalizumab is 11 days, it might be reasonable to hold PLEX in patients diagnosed with PML after a period of time corresponding to more than 5 half-lives of the drug.

IRIS occurrence is usually reported as soon as the effect of Natalizumab is suppressed, when the inflammation recurs again in the CNS, in consequence of the restored lymphocyte trafficking.

Considering that the immune reconstitution can be dramatic, it is important for the clinician to take care of the possibility of fast deterioration of clinical conditions. In this scenario, it is conceivable to get the availability of intensive care support.

Currently, the cardinal therapy for IRIS in the Natalizumab-associated PML patient is based on high-dosage steroids (1 g/d of methylprednisolone for 5 days) followed by a prolonged oral taper over 1 to 2 months, favoring reduction of inflammation. The effectiveness of steroid use is supported particularly in the case of catastrophic IRIS, to prevent brain oedema or risk of herniation, when massive inflammation is supposed to contribute to the possible evolution of the disease. However, steroid use is anecdotal and treatment trials are lacking.

In the case series of Tan et. al, steroid use following the development of IRIS was associated with better outcomes in terms of EDSS [47]. The positive effect of this treatment is not observed in the group of patients presenting with late onset of symptoms, probably because the worse outcome is associated in part to the delay in PML diagnosis.

The risk that corticosteroids may block the immune surveillance against JCV re-activation during PML has been discharged. Indeed complications withholding initiation of steroid treatment are too high, considering that IRIS may be fulminant and result in significant mortality and morbidity.

To prevent the development of IRIS, some experts in the field have advocated for the use of corticosteroids at the time of initiation of plasmapheresis to remove Natalizumab. The theoretic disadvantage of this approach is that if all inflammation was completely prevented, the PML lesion would continue to advance, since the immune response is necessary to control the infection. Such prophylactic approaches would be useful if effective antiviral compounds against JCV were available.

Conclusion

The development of PML-IRIS in MS patients treated with Natalizumab is a frequent event. Natalizumab-associated PML is the result of re-activation of latent JCV. IRIS presents as a subacute progression and exacerbation of earlier symptoms of PML within days to a few weeks after PLEX. It is supposed to be a consequence of the drug removal from the bloodstream by plasma exchange favoring a paradoxical response of the restored immune system towards the CNS white matter, also triggered by JCV antigens exposure stimulating lymphocyte activation.

To estimate the risk, the clinical implications and prognosis of IRIS is becoming increasingly a common situation in the clinical setting of natalizumab treated MS patients. Clinicians have to face with the differential diagnosis, particularly considering that neurological dysfunctions may be interpreted as an acute phase of MS rather than the IRIS, with implications on the therapeutic decisions.

The attention is particularly focused on asymptomatic cases of PML, in which lesions can be observed at MRI in the absence of clinical symptoms. In such patients, preventive therapies and a strict follow up will hopefully prevent pathogenic events leading to overt catastrophic neurological damage.

References

[1] Stoll M. 1., Schmidt R. E. Adverse events of desirable gain in immunocompetence: the Immune Restoration Inflammatory Syndromes. *Autoimmun. Rev.,* 2004 Jun.; 3(4):243-9.

[2] McCarthy M., Nath A. Neurologic consequences of the immune reconstitution inflammatory syndrome (IRIS). *Curr. Neurol. Neurosci. Rep.,* 2010; 10:467–475.

[3] Müller M., Wandel S., Colebunders R., Attia S., Furrer H., Egger M.; IeDEA Southern and Central Africa. Immune reconstitution inflammatory syndrome in patients starting antiretroviral therapy for HIV infection: a systematic review and meta-analysis. *Lancet Infect. Dis.*, 2010; 10(4): 251–261.

[4] Meintjes G., Lawn S. D., Scano F., et al., for the International Network for the Study of HIV-associated IRIS. Tuberculosis-associated immune

reconstitution inflammatory syndrome: case definitions for use in resource-limited settings. *Lancet Infect. Dis.*, 2008; 8: 516–23.

[5] Shelburne I. S. A., Darcourt J., White A. C. Jr., et al. The role of immune reconstitution inflammatory syndrome in AIDS-related Cryptococcus neoformans disease in the era of highly active antiretroviral therapy. *Clin. Infect. Dis.,* 2005; 40: 1049–52.

[6] DeSimone J. A., Pomerantz R. J., Babinchak T. J. Inflammatory reactions in HIV-1-infected persons after initiation of highly active antiretroviral therapy. *Ann. Intern. Med.*, 2000; 133: 447–54.

[7] French M. A. HIV/AIDS: immune reconstitution inflammatory syndrome: a reappraisal. *Clin. Infect. Dis.*, 2009; 48: 101–07.

[8] Dhasmana D., Keertan D., Pernille R., Wilkinson R., Meintjes G. Immune reconstitution inflammatory syndrome in HIV-infected patients receiving antiretroviral therapy. *Drugs,* 2008; 68:191–208.

[9] Pound M. W., May D. B.: Proposed mechanisms and preventative options of Jarisch-Herxheimer reactions. *J. Clin. Pharm. Ther.,* 2005, 30:291–295.

[10] Holzheimer R. G.: Antibiotic induced endotoxin release and clinical sepsis: a review. *J. Chemother.*, 2001, 13 Spec. No 1:159–172.

[11] Pruitt A. A., Graus F., Rosenfeld M. R. Neurological Complications of Solid Organ Transplantation. *The Neurohospitalist*, 2013; 3(3):152-166.

[12] Tan C. S., Koralnik I. J. Progressive multifocal leukoencephalopathy and other disorders caused by JC virus: clinical features and pathogenesis. *Lancet Neurol.*, 2010 Apr.; 9(4):425-37.

[13] Jensen P. N., Major E. O. A classification scheme for human polyomavirus JCV variants based on the nucleotide sequence of the noncoding regulatory region. *J. Neurovirol.*, 2001; 7: 280–87.

[14] Koralnik I. J., Du Pasquier R. A., Letvin N. L. JC virus-specific cytotoxic T lymphocytes in individuals with progressive multifocal leukoencephalopathy. *J. Virol.*, 2001; 75: 3483–7.

[15] Bellizzi A., Anzivino E., Rodio D. M., Palamara A. T., Nencioni L., Pietropaolo V. New insights on human polyomavirus JC and pathogenesis of progressive multifocal leukoencephalopathy. *Clin. Dev. Immunol.*, 2013: 839719.

[16] Whiteman M. L., Post M. J., Berger J. R., Tate L. G., Bell M. D., Limonte LP. Progressive multifocal leukoencephalopathy in 47 HIV-seropositive patients: neuroimaging with clinical and pathologic correlation. *Radiology*, 1993; 187: 233–40.

[17] Sahraian M. A., Radue E. W., Eshaghi A., Besliu S., Minagar A. Progressive multifocal leukoencephalopathy: a review of the neuroimaging features and differential diagnosis. *Eur. J. Neurol.*, 2012 Aug.; 19(8):1060-9.

[18] Astrom K. E., Mancall E. L., Richardson E. P. Jr. Progressive multifocal leuko-encephalopathy; a hitherto unrecognized complication of chronic lymphatic leukaemia and Hodgkin's disease. *Brain*, 1958; 81:93–111.

[19] Berger J. R., Aksamit A. J., Clifford D. B., Davis L., Koralnik I. J., Sejvar J. J., Bartt R., Major E. O., Nath A. PML diagnostic criteria: consensus statement from the AAN Neuroinfectious Disease Section. *Neurology*, 2013 Apr. 9; 80(15): 1430-8.

[20] Mazda M. E., Brosch J. R., Wiens A. L., Bonnin J. M., Kamer A. P., Mattson D. H., et al. A case of natalizumab-associated progressive multifocal leukoencephalopathy with repeated negative CSF JCV testing. *Int. J. Neurosci.*, 2013; 123: 353–7.

[21] Marzocchetti A., Tompkins T., Cliff ord D. B., et al. Determinants of survival in progressive multifocal leukoencephalopathy. *Neurology,* 2009; 73: 1551–58.

[22] Yiannoutsos C. T., Major E. O., Curfman B., et al. Relation of JC virus DNA in the cerebrospinal fl uid to survival in acquired immunodeficiency syndrome patients with biopsy-proven progressive multifocal leukoencephalopathy. *Ann. Neurol.,* 1999; 45: 816–21.

[23] De Luca A., Ammassari A., Pezzotti P., et al. Cidofovir in addition to antiretroviral treatment is not effective for AIDS-associated progressive multifocal leukoencephalopathy: a multicohort analysis. *AIDS*, 2008; 22: 1759–67.

[24] Hall C. D., Dafni U., Simpson D., et al. Failure of cytarabine in progressive multifocal leukoencephalopathy associated with human immunodeficiency virus infection. AIDS Clinical Trials Group 243 Team. *N. Engl. J. Med.,* 1998; 338: 1345–51.

[25] Brickelmaier M. 1., Lugovskoy A., Kartikeyan R., Reviriego-Mendoza M. M., Allaire N., Simon K., Frisque R. J., Gorelik L. Identification and characterization of mefloquine efficacy against JC virus in vitro. *Antimicrob Agents Chemother.*, 2009 May; 53(5):1840-9.

[26] Assetta B. 1., Maginnis M. S., Gracia Ahufinger I., Haley S. A., Gee G. V., Nelson C. D., O'Hara B. A., Allen Ramdial S. A., Atwood W. J. 5-HT2 receptors facilitate JC polyomavirus entry. *J. Virol.,* 2013 Dec.; 87 (24):13490-8.

[27] https://biogenidec.com

[28] Bozic C., Richman S., Plavina T., et al. Anti-JCV antibody prevalence in patients with relapsing multiple sclerosis receiving or considering treatment with natalizumab: baseline results of STRATIFY-2. *Neurology*, 2012; 78.

[29] Dong-Si T., Richman S., Wattjes M. P., Wenten M., Gheuens S., Philip J., Datta S., McIninch J., Bozic C., Bloomgren G., Richert N. Outcome and survival of asymptomatic PML in natalizumab-treated MS patients. *Ann. Clin. Transl. Neurol.*, 2014 Oct.; 1(10):755-64.

[30] Dong-Si T., Gheuens S., Gangadharan A., Wenten M., Philip J., McIninch J., Datta S., Richert N., Bozic C., Bloomgren G., Richman S., Weber T., Clifford D. B. Predictors of survival and functional outcomes in natalizumab-associated progressive multifocal leukoencephalopathy. *J. Neurovirol.*, 2015 Mar. 14.

[31] Chalkley J. J., Berger J. R. Progressive multifocal leukoencephalopathy in multiple sclerosis. *Curr. Neurol. Neurosci. Rep.*, 2013 Dec.; 13(12): 408.

[32] Sereti I., Rodger A. J., French M. A. Biomarkers in immune reconstitution inflammatory syndrome: signals from pathogenesis. *Curr. Opin. HIV AIDS*, 2010 Nov.; 5(6): 504-10.

[33] Antonelli L. R., Mahnke Y., Hodge J. N., et al. Elevated frequencies of highly activated CD4+ T cells in HIV+ patients developing immune reconstitution inflammatory syndrome. *Blood,* 2010; 116:3818–3827.

[34] Price P., Morahan G., Huang D., et al. Polymorphisms in cytokine genes define subpopulations of HIV-1 patients who experienced immune restoration diseases. *AIDS,* 2002; 16:2043–2047.

[35] Stüve O., Marra C. M., Jerome K. R., Cook L., Cravens P. D., Cepok S., et al. Immune surveillance in multiple sclerosis patients treated with natalizumab. *Ann. Neurol.*, (2006) 59(5):743–7.

[36] Reid C. E., Li H., Sur G., Carmillo P., Bushnell S., Tizard R., et al. Sequencing and analysis of JC virus DNA from natalizumab-treated PML patients. *J. Infect. Dis.,* (2011) 204(2):237–44.

[37] Weber T., Trebst C., Frye S., Cinque P., Vago L., Sindic C. J., Schulz-Schaeffer W. J., Kretzschmar H. A., Enzensberger W., Hunsmann G., Luke W. Analysis of the systemic and intrathecal humoral immune response in progressive multifocal leukoencephalopathy. *J. Infect. Dis.,* (1997); 176:250–254.

[38] Weber F., Goldmann C., Kramer M., et al. Cellular and humoral immune response in progressive multifocal leukoencephalopathy. *Ann. Neurol.,* 2001; 49: 636–42.

[39] Du Pasquier R. A., Clark K. W., Smith P. S., et al. JCV-specific cellular immune response correlates with a favorable clinical outcome in HIV-infected individuals with progressive multifocal leukoencephalopathy. *J. Neurovirol.*, 2001; 7:318 –322.

[40] Metz I., Radue E. W., Oterino A., Kümpfel T., Wiendl H., Schippling S., Kuhle J., Sahraian M. A., Gray F., Jakl V., Häusler D., Brück W. Pathology of immune reconstitution inflammatory syndrome in multiple sclerosis with natalizumab-associated progressive multifocal leukoencephalopathy. *Acta Neuropathol.*, 2012 Feb.; 123 (2): 235-45.

[41] Krumbholz M., Meinl I., Kumpfel T., Hohlfeld R., Meinl E. Natalizumab disproportionately increases circulating pre-B and B cells in multiple sclerosis. *Neurology,* (2008) 71:1350–1354.

[42] Chen Y., Bord E., Tompkins T., et al. Asymptomatic reactivation of JC virus in patients treated with natalizumab. *N. Engl. J. Med.,* 2009; 361:1067–1074.

[43] Major E. O., Frohman E., Douek D. JC Viremia in Natalizumab-Treated Patients with Multiple Sclerosis. *The New England journal of medicine,* 2013; 368(23):2240-2241.

[44] McCarthy M., Nath A. Neurologic consequences of the immune reconstitution inflammatory syndrome (IRIS). *Curr. Neurol. Neurosci. Rep.*, 2010 Nov.; 10(6):467-75.

[45] Yousry T. A., Pelletier D., Cadavid D., Gass A., Richert N. D., Radue E. W., Filippi M. Magnetic resonance imaging pattern in natalizumab-associated progressive multifocal leukoencephalopathy. *Ann. Neurol.,* 2012 Nov.; 72(5):779-87.

[46] Blinkenberg M., Sellebjerg F., Leffers A. M., et al. Clinically PML and prolonged immune reconstitution inflammatory syndrome in a patient with multiple sclerosis treated with natalizumab. *Mult. Scler.,* 2013; 19: 1226–1229.

[47] Tan I. L., McArthur J. C., Clifford D. B., Major E. O., Nath A. Immune reconstitution inflammatory syndrome in natalizumab-associated PML. *Neurology,* 2011; 77(11):1061-1067.

[48] Khoury M. N., Alsop D. C., Agnihotri S. P., Pfannl R., Wuthrich C., Ho M. L., Hackney D., Ngo L., Anderson M. P., Koralnik I. J. Hyperintense cortical signal on magnetic resonance imaging reflects focal leukocortical encephalitis and seizure risk in progressive multifocal leukoencephalopathy. *Ann. Neurol.*, 2014 May; 75(5):659-69.

[49] Dahlhaus S., Hoepner R., Chan A., Kleiter I., Adams O., Lukas C., Hellwig K., Gold R. Disease course and outcome of 15 monocentrically

treated natalizumab-associated progressive multifocal leukoencephalopathy patients. *J. Neurol. Neurosurg. Psychiatry*, 2013 Oct.; 84(10):1068-74.

[50] Vermersch P., Kappos L., Gold R., et al. Clinical outcomes of natalizumab-associated progressive multifocal leukoencephalopathy. *Neurology,* 2011; 76:1697–1704.

[51] Calvi A., De Riz M., Pietroboni A. M., Ghezzi L., Maltese V., Arighi A., Fumagalli G. G., Jacini F., Donelli C., Comi G., Galimberti D., Scarpini E. Partial recovery after severe immune reconstitution inflammatory syndrome in a multiple sclerosis patient with progressive multifocal leukoencephalopathy. *Immunotherapy*, 2014; 6(1):23-8.

[52] O'Connor P. W., Goodman A., Kappos L., Lublin F. D., Miller D. H., Polman C., Rudick R. A., Aschenbach W., Lucas N. Disease activity return during natalizumab treatment interruption in patients with multiple sclerosis. *Neurology,* 2011 May 31; 76(22):1858-65.

[53] Khatri B. O., Man S., Giovannoni G., et al. Effect of plasma exchange in accelerating natalizumab clearance and restoring leukocyte function. *Neurology,* 2009; 72:402– 409.

INDEX

F

G

H

I

J

K

L

M

Q

R

S

T